*Colour* Aids

D0713359

# Nephrology

## J. L. Anderton FRCPE

Consultant Nephrologist, Western General
Hospital, Edinburgh

## D. Thomson FRCSE MRCPE FRCPath

Senior Lecturer, Department of Pathology,
University of Edinburgh; Honorary Consultant,
Lothian Health Board

04

Churchill Livingstone

EDINBURGH LONDON MELBOURNE AND NEW YORK 1988

# Preface

This book is intended for medical students and junior medical staff wishing to obtain a basic understanding of clinical nephrology and associated pathological abnormalities. Pathological and clinical features have been collated throughout.

We gratefully acknowledge the kind permission of colleagues who have allowed us to reproduce photographs from their collections.

Edinburgh 1988                                                    J.L.A.
                                                                  D.T.

# Contents

# 1 | Normal Structure: Glomerulus

Each kidney contains around one million glomeruli. The glomerulus consists of a tuft of capillaries functioning at high pressure being interposed between the afferent and efferent arterioles.

**Mesangium**

Consists of mesangial cells surrounded by an amorphous matrix, containing fine fibrils and tubules. At the hilum, the mesangium is continuous with cells of the juxtaglomerular apparatus (JGA). The mesangium apart from its supportive role also plays an important part in the uptake and transport of particulate matter and immune complexes from the capillary lumina.

**Endothelial cells**

Line each capillary; their fenestrated cytoplasm affords direct communication between the lumen and the inner aspect of the capillary basement membrane by means of pores up to 1 000Å across.

**Glomerular basement membrane (GBM)**

Outlining all capillaries and investing all mesangial regions is a finely fibrillar membrane, 3200–3400Å in width and composed of collagenous and non-collagenous proteins. This is the major filter of the glomerulus and acts as a size and charge-selective barrier. The latter function is dependent upon the anionic charge derived mainly from heparan sulphate.

**Epithelial cells**

On the outer aspect of GBM lie the visceral epithelial cells or podocytes whose foot processes or pedicels rest on the GBM.

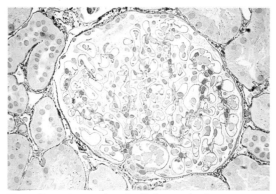

**Fig. 1** Note the paucity of cells in a normal glomerulus. (Haematoxylin and fast green × 200)

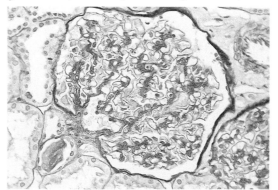

**Fig. 2** Mesangial matrix stained pink shows a branching structure. (PAS × 200)

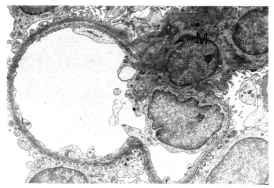

**Fig. 3** A capillary is outlined by the GBM. Pedicels on outer aspect of GBM and note mesangium (M). (× 2700)

## Examination of the urine

**Appearance**

Various changes in colour can occur due to drugs and dyes. Blood will make the urine red or brown.

**Reagent strips**

The reagent strip is dipped into the urine and the colour on each of the squares compared with the colour code on the bottle at the time indicated.
*Protein.* Colour change from yellow (zero) through pale green (1 g/l or $++$) to turquoise (20 g/l or $++++$).
*Glucose.* Light blue (negative) through green (14 mmol/l, $+$) to brown (111 mmol/l, $++++$).
*Blood, haemoglobin and myoglobin.* Orange (negative) through pale green to dark green (large amount).

**24 hour collection**

Obtained for accurate estimation of protein excretion and creatinine concentration (see Creatinine clearance, p. 5). Normal urine contains $< 0.3$ g/24 h of protein.

**Microscopy**

Urine is centrifuged and examined for red and white blood cells. Normal urine contains occasional red and white blood cells and no casts. The urine of patients with glomerulonephritis contains many hyaline, granular and red blood cell casts.

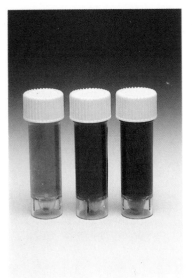

**Fig. 4** Left to right: normal urine; urine containing blood; urine discoloured from patient taking phenolphthalein as laxative.

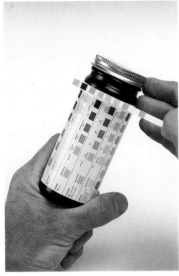

**Fig. 5** Reagent strip test on urine from patient with glomerulonephritis, positive for blood and protein.

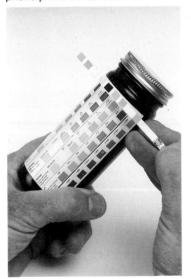

**Fig. 6** Reagent strip from patient with nephrotic syndrome secondary to diabetes mellitus, showing glucose and protein.

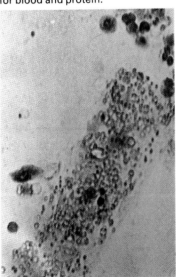

**Fig. 7** Microscopy of urine from patient with glomerulonephritis, showing granular cast.

## Renal function

**Blood tests**

Blood urea and creatinine are routinely measured to give an approximate assessment of renal function. Blood urea is affected by dietary protein and catabolism. Creatinine is less affected by these factors and is a more reliable indicator of renal function.

Normal values:

Blood urea—3–6 mmol/l

Creatinine—60–110 mmol/l

Electrolytes—sodium, potassium and bicarbonate are affected in various renal conditions, e.g. in acute renal failure there is hyperkalaemia and acidosis.

Calcium, phosphate and alkaline phosphatase should be measured when renal bone disease is suspected.

Plasma proteins are assessed in nephrotic patients. Immunological assessment is often required, e.g. anti-nuclear factor (ANF), anti-DNA antibody, complement (C3 and C4).

**Glomerular filtration rate (GFR)**

This function is routinely assessed by creatinine clearance. A 24 h urine collection is made and a blood sample collected during this period.

Creatinine clearance =

$$\frac{\text{Urinary creatinine} \times \text{Volume of urine (ml/min)}}{\text{Plasma creatinine}}$$

Normal value = 124 ± 26 ml/min for adult males and 109 ± 13 ml/min for adult females.

Function declines with renal failure to very low values in acute renal failure and end-stage chronic renal failure.

GFR can also be measured using inulin, $^{51}$Cr-EDTA, $^{125}$I-diatrizoate or $^{125}$I-iothalamate.

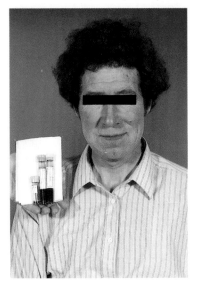

**Fig. 8** Blood samples for urea and electrolytes, creatinine, plasma protein and immunological parameters in patient with glomerulonephritis.

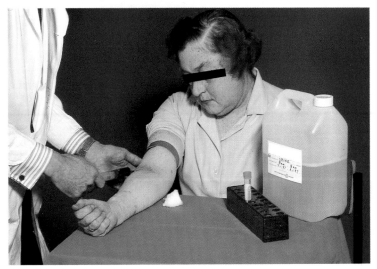

**Fig. 9** 24 h urine collection and blood sample for urinary protein excretion and creatinine clearance measurement in patient with nephrotic syndrome.

# 3 | Radiology of the Kidney (1)

**Plain films**

The whole renal tract—kidney, ureter, bladder (KUB)—is often included in a single plate.
*Kidney size.* In adults the size is 11–15 cm, with no greater difference between right and left than 1.5 cm.
Chronic pyelonephritis, reflux nephropathy, congenital conditions and renal ischaemia cause kidney shrinkage.
Polycystic disease, hydronephrosis and tumours cause enlargement.
*Kidney shape.* Scars may be seen in chronic pyelonephritis. Cysts and tumours cause bulges.
*Calcification.* Stones can be seen in the collecting system. Nephrocalcinosis—calcium in the renal parenchyma—seen in renal tubular acidosis, tuberculosis, and hypercalcaemic states.

**Intravenous urogram (IVU)**

Contrast medium is injected intravenously and films taken of the kidney, ureter and bladder during various phases of function.
*Nephrogram.* Within 1–6 min the renal parenchyma is visualised. At 5–15 min the collecting system including bladder is shown. The patient empties the bladder to assess bladder function. An approximate estimate of kidney function can be made from the density of the nephrogram and the contrast medium in the collecting system. In obstruction the nephrogram phase is prolonged, possibly for hours.
Abnormalities of the collecting system include clubbing of the calyces in chronic pyelonephritis, and dilatation in hydronephrosis (obstruction). Bladder abnormalities can often be identified, e.g. large tumours.

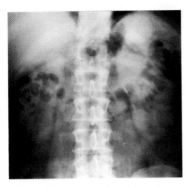

**Fig. 10** Plain X-ray of renal tract (KUB) showing normal kidney size and absence of calculi.

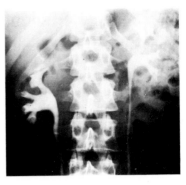

**Fig. 11** Intravenous urogram showing normal calyces, renal pelves and ureters.

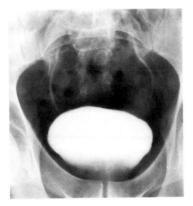

**Fig. 12** Intravenous urogram showing normal bladder.

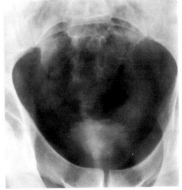

**Fig. 13** Intravenous urogram showing normal emptying of bladder, post-micturition.

# 3 | Radiology of the Kidney (2)

**Cystoureth-rography and retrograde urography**

If detailed information is required about the bladder, cystoscopy is carried out under anaesthesia. The bladder wall can be viewed directly and lesions biopsied, e.g. tumours. If obstruction to the ureter is suspected, a catheter can be passed through the cystoscope into the ureter from the bladder and contrast medium injected.

**Renal angiography**

In severe hypertension which is resistant to treatment, particularly in young patients, stenosis of the renal arteries should be suspected. In these circumstances it is necessary to inject contrast material into the renal arteries via a catheter introduced through the femoral artery.

**Ultrasound**

This is a very convenient method of evaluating the kidneys, ureters and bladder, involving neither injections of contrast media nor the use of ionising radiation. It provides an image which gives anatomical and pathological information. It is of no value in assessing function.
The image of the kidney is shown as follows:
1. The capsule.
2. The cortex separated from the medulla by small arteries.
3. The renal pyramids—echo-free areas within the medulla.
4. The pelvicalyceal system—ovoid collection of dense echoes.
5. The ureters.
6. The bladder.

**Uses**

1. Evidence of obstruction—dilated ureters and pelvicalyceal system.
2. Alteration in size of the kidney, e.g. chronic pyelonephritis, renal artery stenosis.
3. Identification of renal cysts, renal tumours and perinephric collections, e.g. abscess.

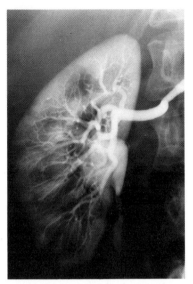

**Fig. 14** Renal angiography showing normal renal arteries and branches.

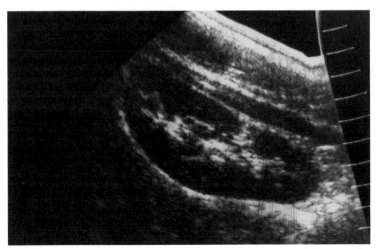

**Fig. 15** Normal ultrasound showing normal renal structure and absence of obstruction.

# 4 | Radio-isotope Studies

Radio-isotopes can be used to assess the anatomy and pathophysiology of the kidney, and the overall or individual renal function. They are useful where poor function or allergy to radiographic contrast material precludes such studies.

**Renogram**

An intravenous bolus of $^{131}$I-orthoiodohippurate or $^{99m}$Tc DTPA technetium is given, the radioactivity counted over each kidney and plotted against time. A curve is obtained with three phases.

1. *Vascular phase.* The sharp upward phase (10–15 s) This corresponds to the appearance of isotope in the kidney.
2. *Secretory phase.* Gradual rise and fall (1–15 min) This corresponds to the secretion of hippurate by the proximal tubules and the passage into the collecting system.
3. *Excretory phase.* (15–30 min) Represents drainage of isotope from the kidney.

The renogram is of particular value in diagnosing renal artery stenosis and urinary obstruction. Micturition urogram can be obtained at the end of this examination to assess the degree of vesico-ureteric reflux.

**Renal scan**

Gamma imaging gives a 'photographic' picture of renal size, shape, position and presence of cysts or tumours. $^{99m}$Tc-DMSA is used which is bound to renal cortex, especially proximal tubules.

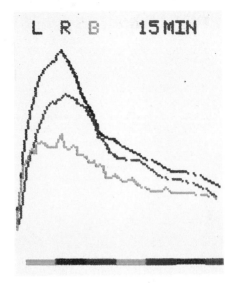

**Fig. 16** Renogram showing vascular, secretory and excretory phases. (L–left; R–right; B–background.)

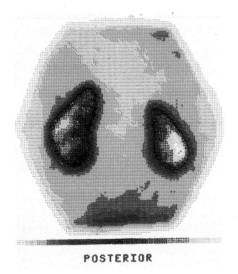

POSTERIOR

**Fig. 17** Renal scan showing normal size and structure of kidneys.

# 5 | Renal Biopsy (Percutaneous)

Renal biopsy is carried out in patients with suspected glomerulonephritis, patients with renal involvement in systemic disease, patients with acute renal failure, and in renal transplant patients with impaired function.

The position of the kidney may be ascertained by previous intravenous urogram or ultrasound.

It is customary to biopsy the right kidney, thus avoiding the spleen.

Contra-indications include any bleeding tendency, severe hypertension, small kidneys, or unilateral kidney.

The patient is placed prone, full antiseptic precautions are taken and local anaesthesia is infused. The lower pole of the kidney is identified using a lumbar puncture needle. The biopsy needle is inserted to the same depth, and a biopsy taken.

The core of renal tissue is divided into 3 pieces, for light microscopy (LM), immunofluorescence (IF) and electron microscopy (EM).

The patient returns to bed and should lie flat for 24 h.

Half hourly pulse and blood pressure measurements are taken for 4 h, hourly readings for a further 4 h and then general observation.

The specimens are sent to the Pathology Department for processing and pathological assessment.

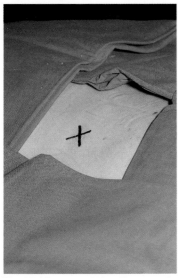

**Fig. 18** Ultrasound identification of lower pole of right kidney.

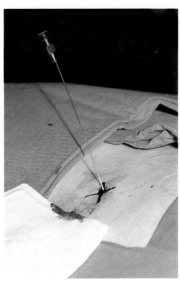

**Fig. 19** Lumbar puncture needle introduced into kidney.

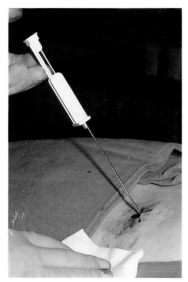

**Fig. 20** Biopsy needle introduced into kidney.

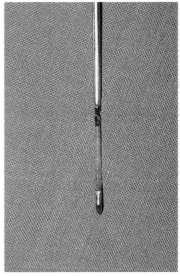

**Fig. 21** Biopsy needle removed containing core of renal tissue.

# 6 | Syndromes of Glomerulonephritis

During the subsequent text, reference is often made to the 'syndromes of glomerulonephritis' which are as follows.

**Acute nephritic syndrome**

A puffy face and small volume of dark urine. The urine contains red cells, red cell casts and a small amount of protein (1–3 g/24 h).
Transient hypertension may occur and the blood urea is occasionally slightly raised.

**Nephrotic syndrome**

This occurs when there is heavy or prolonged proteinuria ($> 4$ g/24 h) resulting in hypoproteinaemia and oedema.

**Acute renal failure**

Occurring when there is a fall in glomerular filtration over a period of a few hours to 2–3 weeks. There is usually oliguria. There is an increase in blood urea and creatinine, a metabolic acidosis, and hyperkalaemia.

**Chronic renal failure**

A syndrome caused by a permanent fall in glomerular filtration rate to values below 10 ml/min, usually progressing over a period of months or years.
Multisystem involvement results in anaemia, hypertension, pericarditis, nausea, diarrhoea, neuropathy, bone disease and finally uraemic coma and death.

**Haematuria, proteinuria, hypertension**

These asymptomatic features may be discovered during routine medical examination, or clinical examination for some other condition and may occur together or alone.

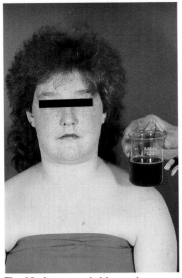

**Fig. 22** Acute nephritic syndrome. Patient with puffy face and smoky urine.

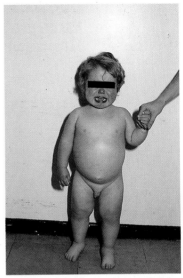

**Fig. 23** Nephrotic syndrome. Child with peripheral oedema, proteinuria and hypoproteinaemia.

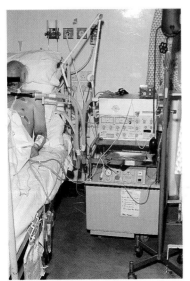

**Fig. 24** Acute renal failure. Patient with oliguria and acute increase in blood urea due to brochopneumonia with septicaemia.

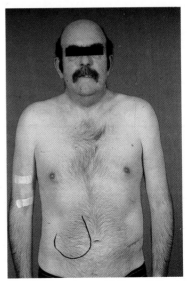

**Fig. 25** Chronic renal failure. Patient with polycystic renal disease (right kidney outlined, left nephrectomy).

# 7 | Diffuse Endocapillary Proliferative Glomerulonephritis (DEPGN)

**Aetiology**

Variable, but may follow an infection after a latent period of 1–2 weeks, particularly beta haemolytic streptococcus (nephritogenic types) affecting throat or skin. Frequently no known cause. Initiated by immune complex deposition or formation in the glomerulus.

**Clinical features**

The common presentation is the acute nephritic syndrome. In the majority, spontaneous remission occurs within 2–3 weeks, although mild haematuria and proteinuria may persist for months.

Occasionally proteinuria is sufficiently marked to cause the nephrotic syndrome.

Acute renal failure requiring dialysis rarely occurs.

About 5 %–10 % progress to chronic renal failure.

**Pathology**

*LM.* All glomeruli enlarged and uniformly hyper-cellular due to marked increase of cells in the mesangium with variable numbers of polymorphs. Capillary lumina are reduced in diameter giving the tuft a solid, bloodless appearance. In severe cases epithelial crescents may be found.

*IF.* Granular deposits of IgG and C3 are found in mesangial and capillary wall sites.

*EM.* The most specific finding is that of large, granular deposits described as 'humps' on the outer aspect of GBM but these usually disappear within a month of the onset.

**Management**

Treat the infection if known, e.g. penicillin for streptococcus, diuretics and anti-hypertensive agents if indicated.

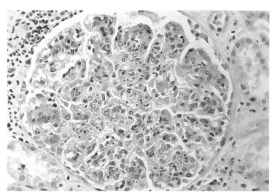

**Fig. 26** Markedly hypercellular including polymorphs producing a solid tuft. (H & E × 200)

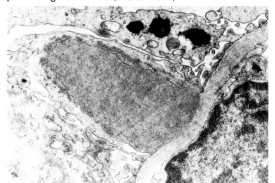

**Fig. 27** Large 'hump' deposit on GBM in post-streptococcal GN. (× 7 200)

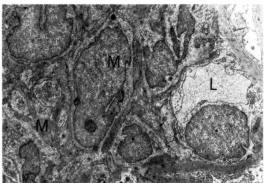

**Fig. 28** Proliferating cells in mesangium (M) encroaching on capillary lumen (L). (× 2 565)

# 8 | Mesangial Proliferative Glomerulonephritis (MPGN)

**Aetiology**

May follow an infective illness but is often of unknown cause. In some instances the lesion may be part of a systemic disease, e.g. SLE.

**Clinical features**

Usually affects children and young adults. Proteinuria and/or haematuria, with or without the nephrotic syndrome is the common presentation. A small percentage progress to chronic renal failure, usually over a number of years.

**Pathology**

*LM.* All glomeruli involved, often to a variable degree, by a minor to moderate increase of cells in the mesangium, usually with a prominent increase in mesangial matrix. Polymorphs are not normally seen in excess numbers and capillary lumina are widely patent.
*IF.* This technique yields a varied pattern which allows for differential diagnosis in some instances. For example, mesangial IgA deposits indicate IgA nephropathy, while IgG, IgM, C3 and C4 on capillary walls can be seen in SLE.
*EM.* Only the presence of dark, granular deposits beneath the GBM overlying the mesangium is distinctive, being seen in cases of IgA nephropathy.

**Management**

Similar to diffuse endocapillary glomerulonephritis.

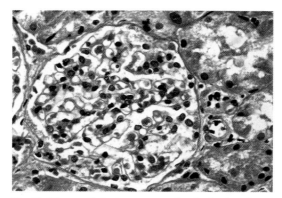

**Fig. 29** Minor cellular increase, no luminal narrowing. (H & E × 200)

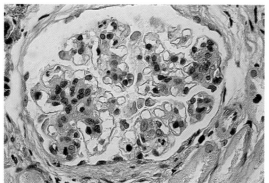

**Fig. 30** Excess of mesangial matrix (stained blue). (Martius Scarlet Blue (MSB) × 200)

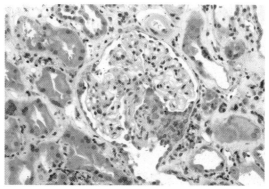

**Fig. 31** Small crescent at 6 o'clock. (H & E × 120)

# 9 | Crescentic Glomerulonephritis (CGN) (Rapidly Progressive Glomerulonephritis)

**Aetiology**

Both anti-glomerular basement membrane antibodies and other immune mechanisms have been implicated. When the basement membrane of the lung is also affected this is called Goodpasture's syndrome.

**Clinical features**

Any age group can be affected. Any or all of the 5 glomerulonephritis syndromes (see p. 15) can be exhibited. Characteristically an acute nephritic illness is followed over a period of weeks by progressive renal failure ending in 1–3 months with chronic renal failure. Haemoptysis in Goodpasture's syndrome.

**Pathology**

*LM.* The diagnostic feature is the finding of epithelial crescents in 70 % or more of the glomeruli. The glomerulus may show changes warranting a second diagnostic label, e.g. DEPGN or MCGN. Thus a crescentic phase, indicative of severe glomerular injury, may be imposed on any underlying pattern. Acute tubular necrosis is a frequent accompaniment of this lesion.
*IF.* 15–20 % of CGN biopsies show linear staining to IgG, indicating anti-GBM disease, mostly as part of Goodpasture's syndrome. Others, however, may be negative save for fibrin in crescents.
*EM.* There are few specific features to be seen apart from identifying the cellular crescent and breaks in GBM.

**Management**

Plasmaphoresis, steroids, and cyclophosphamide.

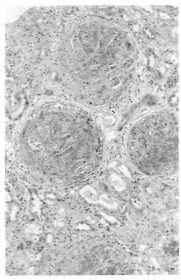

**Fig. 32** Three glomeruli compressed by large crescents. (H & E × 80)

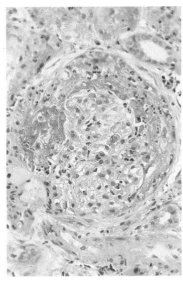

**Fig. 33** Fibrin present in crescent. (MSB × 200)

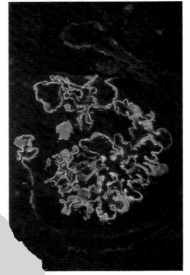

inear staining of IgG in anti-
:ase. (Anti-IgG × 200)

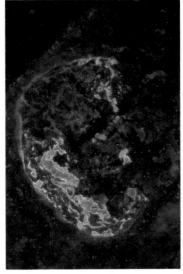

**Fig. 35** Fibrin in crescent; none in glomerulus. (Anti-fibrin × 200)

# Mesangiocapillary Glomerulonephritis (MCGN) (1)
## (Membranoproliferative GN)

**Aetiology**

Usually unknown but in Type 1 immune complexes and complement are involved. In Type 2 the alternate complement pathway is activated and a proportion is associated with partial lipodystrophy.

**Clinical features**

Can affect all ages with equal sex distribution. However, tends to occur predominantly in young adults. The most common presenting feature is the nephrotic syndrome although the other glomerulonephritic syndromes can occur. The condition progresses to chronic renal failure within 5–10 years.

Serum C3 levels are reduced in both Types 1 and 2, but the early acting complement compounds C1, C4 and C2 are often normal in Type 2 disease. C3 nephritic factor is found in Type 2. Type 2 is often associated with prolonged hypocomplementaemia.

**Pathology**

*LM.* This is characterised by mesangial hypercellularity and thickening of peripheral capillary walls affecting all glomeruli. There is often an accentuated lobular pattern and, as an index of the severity of the disease process, epithelial crescents may be present. There are two principal sub-types of MCGN, Type 1 and Type 2, which can sometimes be diagnosed on LM by PAS staining.

Type 1 shows double-contouring of the capillary wall, the outer contour being GBM while the inner one is formed by mesangial matrix, interposed between GBM and the endothelium.

Type 2 shows a refractile, thickened ribbon of PAS positive material superimposed upon the GBM. This material also stains bright green with Masson's trichrome and fluoresces with thiofla T.

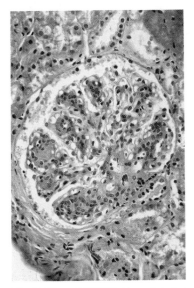

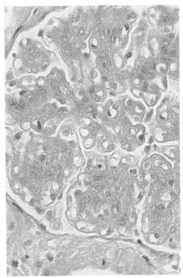

**Fig. 36** Type 1 MCGN: Hyperlobulated tuft with mesangial proliferation and GBM thickening. (H & E × 200)

**Fig. 37** Type 1 MCGN: This shows 'double-contouring'. (MSB × 320)

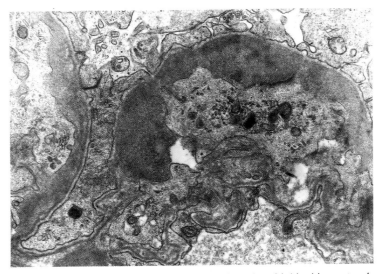

**Fig. 38** Type 1 MCGN: Large subendothelial deposits with 'double-contour' effect. (× 14 250)

# Mesangiocapillary Glomerulonephritis (MCGN) (2)

**Pathology**
(cont)

*IF.* In Type 1 there is usually IgG and C3 both on capillary walls and in mesangium but IgM, C4 and C1q can also be found.

In Type 2 there may be a characteristic pattern of intense granular staining to C3 alone in the mesangium and to a much lesser extent on capillary walls, but frequently IgG, IgM and fibrin are found in addition.

*EM.* Type 1: Granular subendothelial deposits often of a very large size. Variable numbers of subepithelial deposits in a minority of patients. The double contour of GBM and mesangial matrix can be clearly shown.

Type 2: Electron-dense, black deposit overlies most or all of the GBM and is also present in Bowman's capsule and tubular basement membrane (TBM). Similar black deposit in mesangium.

**Management**

No known specific treatment for glomerular lesion. Condition progresses and steroids and immunosuppressive agents have not been shown to be of any value.

Nephrotic syndrome, hypertension and renal failure treated by appropriate measures.

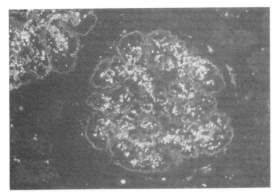

**Fig. 39** Type 2 MCGN: Abundant C3 in mesangium and also on GBM. (Anti-C3 × 200)

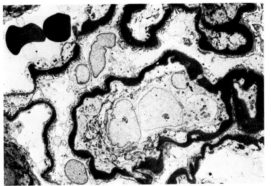

**Fig. 40** Type 2 MCGN: Dense deposit within GBM. (× 1 170)

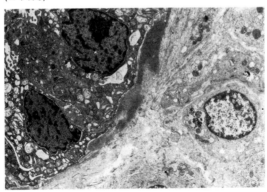

**Fig. 41** Type 2 MCGN: Dense deposit within TBM. (× 3 240)

# 11 | Minimal Lesion Glomerulonephritis

**Aetiology**

No aetiological agent has been identified. There is some evidence to suggest immunological deficiency. Patients with atopic features seem predisposed to develop this condition and abnormalities in T cell function have been noted.

**Clinical features**

Classically presents as the nephrotic syndrome in children and young adults. Proteinuria is highly selective.

**Pathology**

*LM.* Glomeruli are of normal size and cellularity; GBM not altered. Some workers would accept a minimal increase in mesangial cells under this heading, and such cases, certainly in childhood, behave no differently to those showing no hypercellularity.
*IF.* Most cases are negative for Ig and C; some show faint capillary wall (or mesangial) staining for IgM and C3, of doubtful significance.
*EM.* The most obvious change is the widespread loss of pedicels, the outer aspect of the GBM being invested with a thin rim of epithelial cytoplasm. The GBM itself is of normal appearance, devoid of deposits. Both fibrin and platelets have been found in capillary lumina in 5–10 % of cases presumed to be a reflection of hypovolaemia and hyperviscosity.
In remission, pedicel structure is rapidly reconstituted.

**Management**

Good response to steroids and, if resistant or persistent relapse, give cyclophosphamide.

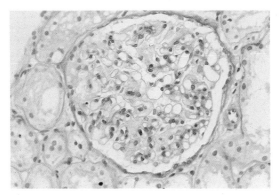

**Fig. 42** Glomerulus appears normal on light microscopy. (H & E × 200)

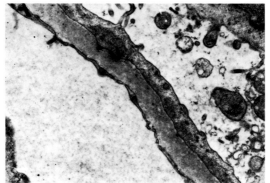

**Fig. 43** GBM of normal width with no deposits. Total loss of pedicels. (× 9 000)

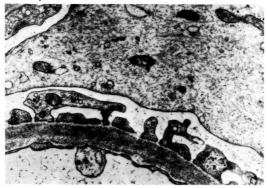

**Fig. 44** In remission, pedicels promptly restored. (× 9 000)

# 12 | Membranous Glomerulonephritis (MGN)

**Aetiology**

In the majority of cases there is no known aetiological factor. Immune deposits are seen but their origin remains obscure. In a minority of cases other factors are implicated: neoplastic disease with immune complexes involving tumour antigens; infections—hepatitis B and malaria; drugs—penicillamine, gold, possibly organic solvents.

**Clinical features**

Adults, any age, male predominance.
The majority present with nephrotic syndrome. A few present with asymptomatic proteinuria and haematuria, and some with chronic renal failure. About 25 % go into spontaneous remission.

**Pathology**

*LM.* Uniform increase in the width of GBM affecting all glomeruli without any significant hypercellularity. In early cases methenamine silver impregnation displays a characteristic spike pattern on the outer aspect of the GBM, the spikes representing shoulders of basement membrane material cupping immune deposits.
*IF.* IgG and C3 are deposited on the outer side of the GBM in a continuous, beaded pattern.
*EM.* In the early stages, large numbers of granular subepithelial deposits can be found overlying a GBM which, apart from the protruding spikes, is of normal thickness. Pedicel structure is largely effaced. Later GBM becomes irregularly thickened, spikes are lost and partly or wholly translucent deposits are incorporated within the GBM.

**Management**

High dose steroids on alternate days for 3 months.

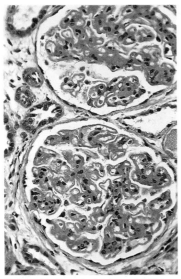

**Fig. 45** Uniformly thickened GBM, no proliferation. (H & E × 200)

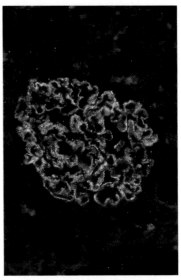

**Fig. 46** Granular deposits of IgG on thickened GBM. (Anti-IgG × 200)

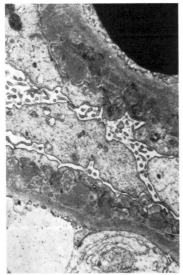

**Fig. 47** Granular and partly lucent deposits on outer aspect of GBM. Pedicels lost. (× 12 600)

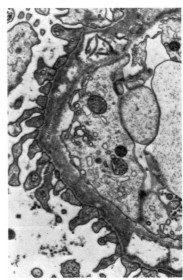

**Fig. 48** Lucent deposits now on inner aspect of GBM and pedicels reformed in remission. (× 9 000)

# 13 | Focal and Segmental Proliferative Glomerulonephritis (FGN)

**Aetiology**

In many cases this remains obscure. The condition is sometimes associated with non-specific infection and systemic disease such as systemic lupus erythematosus.

**Clinical features**

The most common presenting feature is haematuria. Proteinuria is minimal and the nephrotic syndrome rarely encountered. The prognosis is generally good but some progress to renal impairment.

**Pathology**

*LM.* The critical diagnostic feature is that the cellular proliferation affects only a small percentage of the glomeruli, the majority being normal—hence 'focal'. Even those tufts which are hypercellular may frequently show changes affecting some lobules but not others—'segmental'.

*IF.* A variety of patterns can be seen in FGN depending upon the underlying cause. In IgA disease or Henoch-Schonlein syndrome a diffuse mesangial deposition of granular IgA, often with IgG and C3, is seen. In SLE any or all of the Igs may be present, as well as early and late reacting C components, and these are on GBM as well as in mesangium. In cases of polyarteritis however, there is usually no fluorescence or, at most, there are focal deposits of fibrin. Thus IF findings may help in making a definitive diagnosis.

*EM.* IgA nephropathy and SLE show features listed elsewhere; otherwise no diagnostic lesions are seen.

**Management**

Usually no specific treatment but if systemic diseases, e.g. SLE, use steroids.

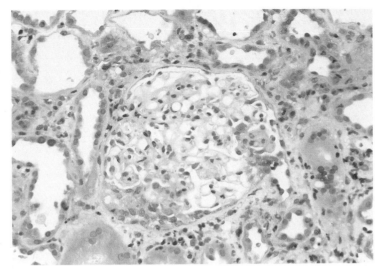

**Fig. 49** Segmental proliferation at 4 o'clock and small crescent at 7 o'clock. (H & E × 280)

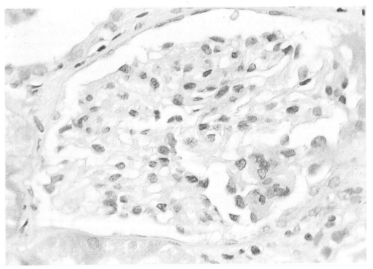

**Fig. 50** Proliferation involving the lobule at 4 o'clock. (H & E × 448)

# 14 | Focal and Segmental Glomerulosclerosis (FSG)
## (Focal Hyalinosis)

**Aetiology**

This remains obscure. There may be an overlap between minimal lesion glomerulonephritis and FSG.

**Clinical features**

Children and adults.
Often presents as nephrotic syndrome.
Occasionally picked up as asymptomatic haematuria and proteinuria. Most cases progress to chronic renal failure over 10–15 years.

**Pathology**

*LM.* Early in the disease most glomeruli are normal but some show segmental sclerosis of the tuft. In addition deposits of hyaline, PAS positive material are seen both in sclerotic areas and as isolated lesions in capillary lumina. Most cases show no hypercellularity but some show a mild diffuse increase of mesangial cells.
The proportion of sclerotic areas increases and finally involves whole glomeruli—global sclerosis—heralding the onset of renal failure.
*IF.* IgM and C3 are found in sclerotic foci.
*EM.* Sclerotic foci show wrinkling of GBM, increase of mesangial matrix and local effacement of pedical structure. Electron-dense deposits are found in relation to areas of hyalinosis.

**Management**

There is no response to steroids or immunosuppression.

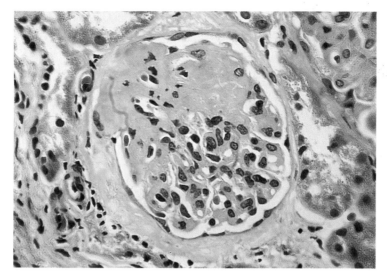

**Fig. 51** Sclerotic focus in upper half of glomerulus. (H & E × 280)

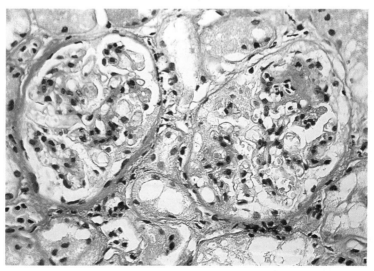

**Fig. 52** Single sclerotic focus in tuft on the right otherwise both glomeruli normal. (MSB × 280)

# 15 | Systemic Lupus Erythematosus

**Aetiology**

Anti-nuclear antibodies form autoimmune complexes which are deposited in glomerular capillaries. Precipitating factors include viral infection, genetic predisposition, and drugs, e.g. hydrallazine.

**Clinical features**

Onset predominantly at ages 20–30, women more than men. Multisystem involvement. Erythematous rash over exposed areas, arthritis, pericarditis and valvular disease, pleurisy, liver failure, epilepsy and neurological deficits, anaemia, thrombocytopenia. Renal involvement may present as any of the 5 glomerulonephritis syndromes (see p. 15). Immunological abnormalities: reduced C3 and C4; anti-nuclear antibodies to DNA and RNA and double-stranded DNA are present.

**Pathology**

*LM.* A variety of patterns may be seen in SLE. The commonest is DEPGN (45 %) followed by MPGN (20 %), FGN (20 %) and MGN (15 %). Small numbers of cases show MCGN and most can show, in addition, crescents to a varying degree. The finding of crescents and/or foci of necrosis indicates an active florid lesion. In such cases intracapillary thrombi and haemotoxylin bodies can often be found.
*IF.* Frequently a 'full house' of immunoglobulins, IgG, IgM, C3, C4 and Clq, and fibrin will be seen in a granular fashion on the thickened GBM.
*EM.* Large, dark granular deposits on both sides of and within the GBM are strongly suggestive of SLE. However, deposits may be restricted to the subendothelial aspect of GBM or, as in the MGN pattern, the subepithelial aspect.

**Management**

Steroids, sometimes supplemented by azathioprine or cyclophosphamide. Appropriate management for nephrotic syndrome, acute and chronic renal failure.

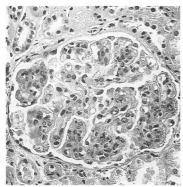

**Fig. 53** Diffuse proliferation and focal GBM thickening. (H & E × 200)

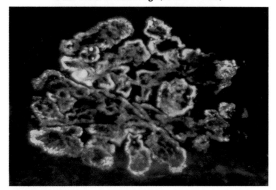

**Fig. 54** Abundant IgG mainly on capillary walls. (Anti IgG × 200)

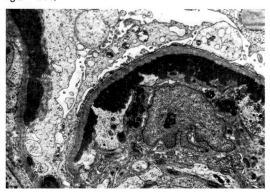

**Fig. 55** Abundant dark deposit on both sides of the GBM. (× 2475)

# 16 | Polyarteritis

**Aetiology**

Unknown, but a hypersensitivity phenomenon associated with immune complex deposition in vessels of various sizes is involved. Hepatitis B associated antigen implicated in some cases.

**Clinical features**

Older males most common.
*Renal manifestations.* Any of the 5 glomerulonephritis syndromes. Nephrotic syndrome is a common presenting feature, and many cases progress to chronic renal failure.

1. *Classic polyarteritis.* Multisystem involvement with severe hypertension, fever, abdominal pain, coronary artery disease and central nervous system involvement.
2. *Microscopic polyarteritis.* Skin lesions common (e.g. purpura, urticaria), arthropathy, pulmonary features (e.g. asthma, infiltrates, pleural effusions), pericarditis and myocarditis. Renal failure often rapidly progressive. Frequently eosinophilia.

**Pathology**

*LM.* Two distinct patterns can be found:

1. *Classic (large vessel) polyarteritis.* Affects muscular arteries and spares glomeruli. Involved vessels show fibrinoid necrosis, acute inflammation and thrombosis while others may show recanalisation and healing. Therefore, both recent and healed infarcts can be found.
2. *Microscopic polyarteritis.* The most usual lesion is a focal proliferative GN with areas of necrosis. Crescents often present and in some cases may be so plentiful as to warrant the diagnosis of crescentic GN.

*IF.* Usually no components other than fibrin are identified in glomeruli and IgM in arteries.
*EM.* Deposits are found very infrequently.

**Management**

Steroids often in high dose, possibly supplemented by cyclophosphamide.

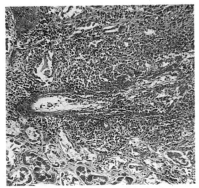

**Fig. 56** In classic polyarteritis the large arteries are involved. (H & E × 80)

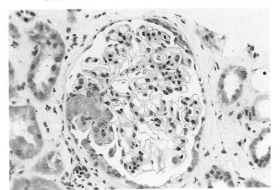

**Fig. 57** Focal necrotising lesion in microscopic polyarteritis. (H & E × 200)

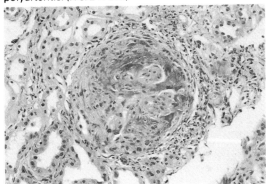

**Fig. 58** Crescentic GN is often seen in microscopic polyarteritis. (MSB × 200)

# 17 | Scleroderma (Systemic Sclerosis)

**Aetiology**

Possible serum cytotoxic factor damages endothelial cells in arteries and capillaries. Vascular permeability leads to overproduction of collagen by fibroblasts.

**Clinical features**

Third to fifth decades. Female : male = 4 : 1. Multisystem involvement. Skin: smooth, thick and stiff. Raynaud's phenomenon and sclerodactyly. Face: smooth, stiff, loss of expression, telangiectases. Subcutaneous calcific deposits (calcinosis). Oesophagus: 'heartburn', regurgitation, dysphagia. Kidneys: progressive renal failure in about half of the cases. Can present with acute renal failure. Nephrotic syndrome occasionally. Severe hypertension is common. Microangiopathic anaemia can occur.

**Pathology**

*LM.* Arterioles and small arteries are the main sites of damage. The former have foci of fibrinoid necrosis and intra-luminal thrombosis while the latter show subintimal accumulation of a loose myxomatous tissue due to acid mucopolysaccharide deposition. Glomeruli may show little change or, in severe cases, focal necrotising lesions may be seen often affecting the vessels at the hilum. Diffuse GBM thickening may occasionally be present.
*IF.* The most consistent finding is of fibrinogen in vessel walls at the sites mentioned above. IgM and C3 may be present also, but inconstantly.
*EM.* There are no distinctive diagnostic findings.

**Management**

Appropriate treatment for hypertension and renal failure.

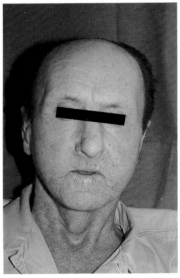

**Fig. 59** Patient with systemic sclerosis showing tight skin over face with telangiectasia.

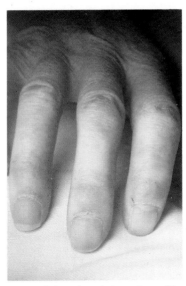

**Fig. 60** Sclerodactyly in patient with systemic sclerosis.

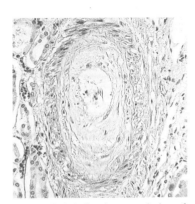

**Fig. 61** Sub-intimal accumulation of pale, myxoid material in interlobular artery. (H & E × 200)

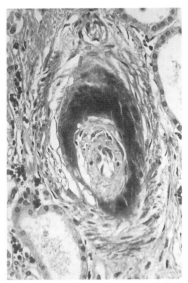

**Fig. 62** Similar vessel stained with PAS (PAS × 200)

# 18 | IgA Nephropathy (Berger's Disease)

**Aetiology**

Usually follows within a day or two of viral upper respiratory tract infection. There is some association between abnormal IgA handling by the liver and gastro-intestinal tract.

**Clinical features**

Occurs in the age group 10–50 years (most common 15–35 years).
Macroscopic haematuria occurs and there may be malaise, loin discomfort and low grade fever. Urinalysis reveals macroscopic and microscopic haematuria and mild proteinuria. Renal function is initially normal but approximately 50 % develop chronic renal insufficiency over a period of years.

**Pathology**

*LM.* The most frequent appearance is of mesangial proliferative glomerulonephritis (MPGN) but in other instances the glomeruli may show focal proliferative glomerulonephritis (FGN) or appear normal.
*IF.* Bright granular deposits of IgA are found throughout the mesangium and less frequently IgG and C3 are seen in the same situation.
*EM.* There is usually a variable increase in mesangial cells and matrix but the most characteristic finding is of dark, granular deposits beneath the basement membrane overlying the mesangium and often within the mesangial matrix.

**Management**

Antibiotics, steroids and immunosuppressive drugs have not been shown to halt the progress of the disease.

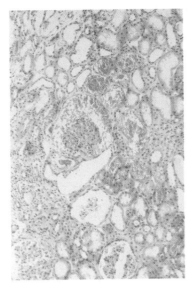

**Fig. 63** Numerous RBCs in Bowman's space and in tubules. (H & E × 80)

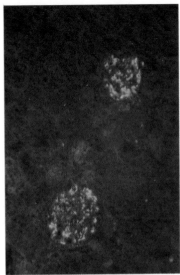

**Fig. 64** IgA present only in glomeruli. (Anti-IgA × 80)

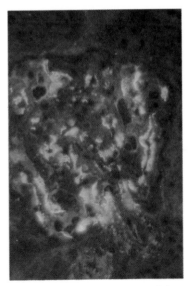

**Fig. 65** This shows the mesangial localisation of the IgA. (Anti-IgA × 200)

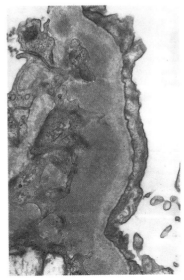

**Fig. 66** Dark, granular deposit beneath GBM overlying mesangium. (× 12 600)

# 19 | Henoch-Schönlein Purpura (HSP)

**Aetiology**

Circulatory cryoglobulins and immune IgA complexes may play a part.
Food allergy and upper respiratory infections possibly involved.

**Clinical features**

Mostly children, males more than females.
Skin: purpura mostly legs and buttocks.
Gut: abdominal pain, haematemesis and melaena.
Joints: diffuse, mild and transient arthritis.
Kidneys: affected in about half cases. Mostly mild involvement with haematuria and mild proteinuria.
Occasionally nephrotic syndrome.
Occasionally acute and/or chronic renal failure, both of which are the major serious complications in HSP.
Serum IgA levels increased in half the cases.

**Pathology**

*LM.* A variety of glomerular lesions may be noted. FGN is the commonest followed by MPGN. The most important features to be assessed, however, are the percentage of crescents and foci of necrosis as prognosis is adversely affected by the presence of either.
*IF.* IgA in a mesangial distribution is almost always seen with IgG and C3 noted in 30–40 %.
*EM.* Electron-dense deposits in mesangium and, in a few cases, on the GBM as well.

**Management**

Analgesics for abdominal and joint pain. Steroids and immunosuppressive agents have been used in acute renal failure, but are of doubtful value.
Appropriate treatment for renal failure.

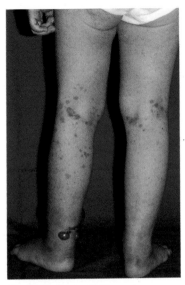

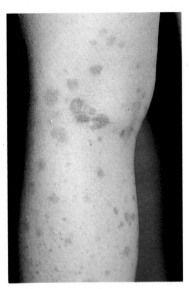

**Fig. 67** Patient with Henoch-Schönlein disease showing purpura over legs.

**Fig. 68** Close-up of purpura.

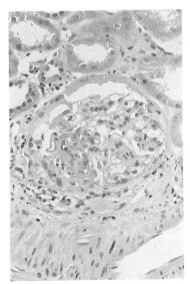

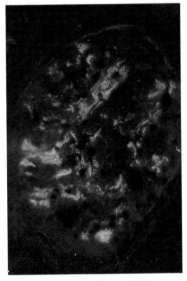

**Fig. 69** Focal proliferation with capsular adhesion. (H & E × 200)

**Fig. 70** Diffuse mesangial IgA deposition. (Anti-IgA × 200)

# 20 | Diabetic Nephropathy

**Aetiology**

Diabetic glomerulosclerosis occurs in both Type 1 insulin-dependent and Type 2 non-insulin-dependent diabetes mellitus. Altered insulin/glucose metabolism affects the mesangium and basement membrane of the glomerular capillaries and tubules, perhaps due to diversion of glucose towards structural pathways.

**Clinical features**

1. Early subclinical proteinuria, only detected by specialised techniques. 2. Nephrotic syndrome. 3. Progressive renal failure. 4. Hypertension. The last three are referred to as the Kimmelstiel-Wilson syndrome. Progression to end-stage renal failure from 4–10 years.

**Pathology**

*LM 1. Diffuse glomerulosclerosis.* There is increased pink, PAS positive material within the mesangium and a fairly uniform increase in thickness of GBM. Progression of the lesion results in an increasingly solid and ultimately wholly sclerosed glomerulus.
*2. Nodular glomerulosclerosis.* The 'nodules' affect one or more lobules in a tuft and consist of a dense, pink, homogenous nodule with a rim of mesangial cells. In addition, fibrin deposits may be seen within capillaries ('exudative lesions') or on Bowman's capsule ('capsular drop'). Arterioles show hyaline change in their media even in the absence of hypertension.
*IF.* IgG and albumin, and less frequently IgM and C3, can often be found, usually in a linear fashion on GBM and also on TBM and Bowman's capsule.
*EM.* The principal findings are an increase of mesangial matrix (including the nodules) and a bland increase in GBM thickness up to 10 times the normal width.

**Management**

Appropriate treatment of hypertension, nephrotic syndrome and chronic renal failure.

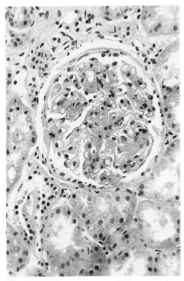

**Fig. 71** Diffuse mesangial sclerosis and prominence of GBM. (H & E × 200)

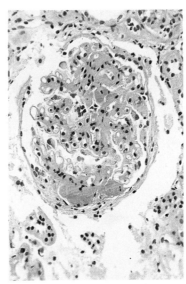

**Fig. 72** Similar plus an exudative lesion at 6 o'clock. (H & E × 200)

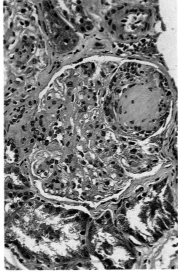

**Fig. 73** Kimmelstiel-Wilson nodule top right. (H & E × 200)

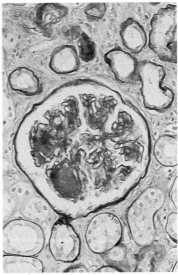

**Fig. 74** PAS stain emphasises GBM thickening, mesangial sclerosis and nodule formation. (PAS × 200)

# 21 | Renal Amyloidosis

**Aetiology**

Extra-cellular deposition of a fibrillar glycoprotein (amyloid). 1. Primary: no known cause. 2. Secondary to (*a*) chronic infection, e.g. osteomyelitis; (*b*) chronic inflammatory conditions, e.g. rheumatoid arthritis; (*c*) neoplastic conditions, e.g. multiple myeloma; (*d*) heredo-familial with Mediterranean fever; (*e*) dialysis—deposition of B2 microglobulin.

**Clinical features**

Multisystem involvement including: waxy plaques or papules in the skin, cardiac failure and dysrythmias, diffuse gastro-intestinal involvement with steatorrhoea, neuropathy, carpal-tunnel syndrome and arthritis.
*Renal features* consist of proteinuria with progression to nephrotic syndrome and chronic renal failure.

**Pathology**

*LM.* Amyloid appears as a pale pink homogenous deposit when stained by H & E. It is initially laid down in the mesangium but later on the GBM also. Accummulation of amyloid leads to progressive replacement of the glomerulus. Amyloid is also to be found in many cases in blood vessel walls and TBM. It is best stained with Congo red (red brown colour) and then viewed under polarised light when the deposits show apple green birefringence.
*IF.* Sometimes negative but Ig and C can be found. On occasion a single heavy and/or light chain may be seen, indicative of a monoclonal origin.
*EM.* This shows numerous short fibrils $1\mu$ in length, with a haphazard arrangement in most instances. Occasionally spike deposits on the outer GBM show a parallel pattern of fibrils.

**Management**

Appropriate treatment for nephrotic syndrome and renal failure. No treatment specifically for amyloid.

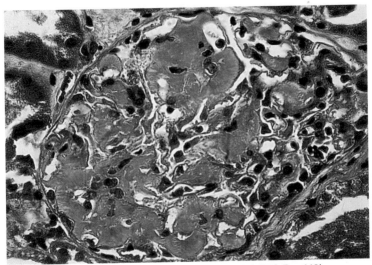

**Fig. 75** Large deposits of pale, pink, hyaline material. (H & E × 448)

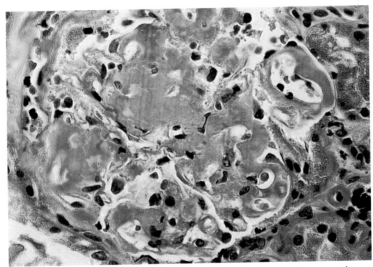

**Fig. 76** These deposits stain reddish-brown with Congo red. (Congo red × 448)

# Nephropathy in Dysproteinaemias (1)

## Multiple myeloma

**Aetiology**

Malignant proliferation of plasma cells producing excessive quantities of monoclonal immunoglobulins which may be deposited in glomerular capillaries. Monoclonal light chains (Bence-Jones protein) are also produced in excess and, because of small size, are filtered and precipitate in tubules forming casts which provoke a cellular reaction.

**Clinical features**

Bone pain (e.g. spine, ribs, skull), anaemia, susceptibility to infection.
Renal features include acute and chronic renal failure. Hypercalcaemia due to bone resorption, hyperuricaemia due to high turnover of nucleoproteins, and amyloidosis contribute to renal deterioration.
Investigation reveals myeloma band on serum electrophoresis, and Bence-Jones (light chain) proteinuria.

**Pathology**

*LM.* The most characteristic lesion is the finding of eosinophilic casts within distal tubules. These provoke proliferation of tubular epithelium and giant cells, probably histiocytic in nature, may be incorporated within the cast. There is often a degree of interstitial oedema and fibrosis. In a few cases (10 %) there may be deposits of amyloid (see p. 47). Deposits of light chains in glomeruli may result in a lobular pattern of glomerulonephritis, 'light chain nephropathy' (LCN), which resembles the Kimmelstiel-Wilson lesion of diabetes.
*EM.* Dark granular deposit is found in the mesangium and on the inner aspect of GBM.
*IF.* Within casts and glomeruli a variety of heavy and light chains can be found. Most usually a monoclonal light chain is present.

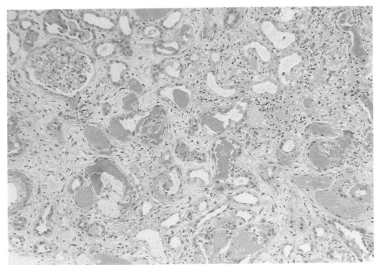

**Fig. 77** Tubular casts in myeloma. (H & E × 112)

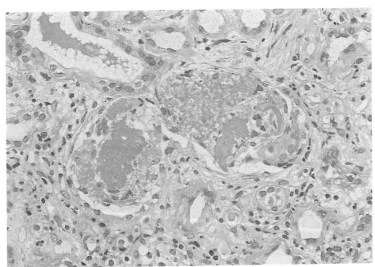

**Fig. 78** The casts provoke a marked cellular response. (H & E × 280)

# Nephropathy in Dysproteinaemias (2)

## Waldenström's macroglobulinaemia

**Aetiology**

Lymphoproliferation produces excessive monoclonal IgM which is deposited in glomerular capillaries.

**Clinical features**

Features of lymphoma. Mild impairment of renal function. Occasionally acute renal failure or nephrotic syndrome. Electrophoresis of plasma shows a monoclonal IgM peak.

**Pathology**

*LM.* Large deposits within glomerular capillaries of hyaline, PAS positive material.
*EM.* These deposits are subendothelial in position.
*IF.* shows deposits to contain IgM and a single light chain. The interstitium contains lymphocytes and plasma cells.

## Mixed cryoglobulinaemia

**Aetiology**

Idiopathic or tumour induced production of IgG-IgM which precipitate in cold. These cryoglobulins deposited in glomerular capillaries.

**Clinical features**

All 5 types of renal presentation associated with vasculitis, purpura, splenomegaly and arthralgia.

**Pathology**

*LM.* Mesangial proliferative or a mesangiocapillary GN. Hyaline deposits in capillary lumina. Arterioles and arteries may show 'arteritic' changes.
*IF.* IgG, IgM and C in glomeruli and arteries/arterioles.
*EM.* Subendothelial deposits with crystalline structure of curved cylinders.

**Management**

Steroids and immunosuppressive drugs may be used in all 3 dysproteinaemias.

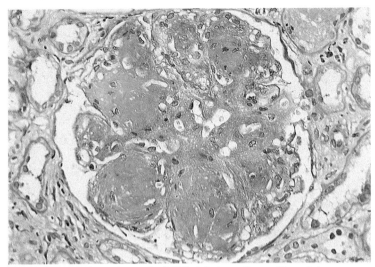

**Fig. 79** Light chain nephropathy (LCN): lobular pattern with nodules reminiscent of diabetes. (PAS × 280)

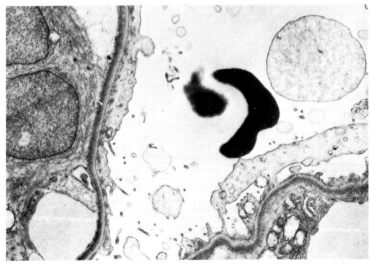

**Fig. 80** LCN: dark, granular deposit on inner half of GBM. RBC in the urinary space. × (5 334)

# 23 | Infective Endocarditis

**Aetiology**

Infection of diseased heart valves (congenital, rheumatic or sclerotic) with micro-organisms (e.g. *Streptococcus viridans, Staphylococcus aureus*, occasionally fungi or rickettsiae) results in formation of antigen antibody immune complexes—deposited in glomerular capillaries and mesangium. Embolisation results in renal infarction and abscess.

**Clinical features**

May be antecedent infection or dental extraction. General malaise, fever, weight loss. Skin: café au lait appearance, petechiae. Fingers: splinter haemorrhages, Osler nodes, clubbing.
Features of the underlying condition are found (e.g. mitral incompetence). The character of the murmur may change.
Renal features are of 2 types.
*1. Emboli. Renal infarction:* loin pain, haematuria; subsequent abscess—fever and general debility.
*2. Immune complex glomerulonephritis.* All 5 types of renal presentation can occur.
Investigations reveal the infecting organism in the blood culture, and the urine contains blood, protein and casts. Circulating immune complexes are present. Echocardiography reveals the nature and progression of the cardiac lesion.

**Pathology**

*LM.* There is commonly a focal proliferative GN, often with necrosis, but diffuse proliferative and mesangiocapillary patterns can be found. In severe cases, crescents will be present with some tubular atrophy/necrosis.
*IF.* Even in the focal form, there is diffuse deposition of IgG, IgM, C3 and fibrin on capillary walls and in the mesangium.
*EM.* Reveals electron-dense deposits in a similar distribution.

**Management**

Intensive appropriate antibiotics. Occasionally valve replacement is necessary. Appropriate management of renal failure.

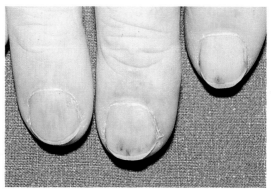

**Fig. 81** Splinter haemorrhages in nails of patient with infective endocarditis.

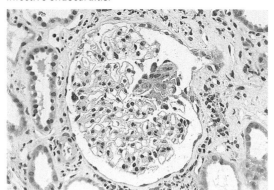

**Fig. 82** Focal proliferation seen at 3 o'clock. (H & E × 200)

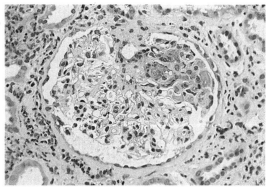

**Fig. 83** Focal proliferation with necrosis. (MSB & 200)

# 24 | Haemolytic Uraemic Syndrome (HUS)

**Aetiology**

Seen in children following viral illness, gastro-intestinal and chest infections.
Features similar to haemolytic uraemic syndrome may be seen in adults with septicaemia, in women on the contraceptive pill or in postpartum renal failure, in malignant hypertension, and associated with severe transplant rejection.

**Clinical features**

Triad of acute renal failure, haemolytic anaemia and thrombocytopenia.
Other features due to intravascular coagulation include: vomiting, haematemesis, malaena; fits, cerebro-vascular accidents, coma.
Raised blood urea, thrombocytopenia, haemolytic anaemia, raised reticulocyte count, deficiency of coagulation factors and raised fibrin degradation products. Helmet cells and burr cells in peripheral blood.
There are similarities between the clinical and pathological features of HUS and thrombotic thrombocytopenic purpura, and disseminated intravascular coagulation.

**Pathology**

*LM.* Fibrin thrombi are found in glomerular capillaries and arterioles. Arteries show intimal thickening and fibrinoid change in their walls. Glomeruli may contain foci of necrosis and there is a variable degree of mesangial hypercellularity. Tubules often show necrosis/atrophy.
*IF.* Fibrin is seen on capillary walls and in the lumen. Ig is an infrequent accompaniment.

**Management**

The efficacy of cortico-steroids and heparin is uncertain. Fresh frozen plasma or purified prostacyclin shows promising results. Dialysis is required if severe renal failure is present. With these measures a favourable outcome is likely. The mortality in children is between 10–20%, however.

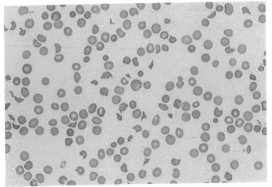

**Fig. 84** A blood film of patient with haemolytic uraemic syndrome showing fragmentation of RBCs.

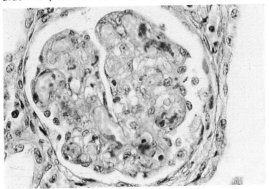

**Fig. 85** Numerous red fibrin thrombi in capillaries. (MSB & 320)

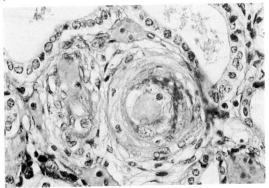

**Fig. 86** Fibrinoid change in vessel wall. (MSB × 320)

# Inherited Glomerulopathies

## Alport's syndrome

**Aetiology**

X-linked with variable penetrance.

**Clinical features**

Haematuria, proteinuria and deafness. Chronic renal failure in males.

**Pathology**

*LM.* Usually a focal or mesangial proliferative GN but crescents may be found. Later, glomerulosclerosis and chronic interstitial nephritis are seen, with interstitial foam cells.
*EM.* GBM may show areas of thinning and of thickening and, as a highly suggestive but not pathognomonic feature, widespread fibrillation and splitting are usually noted—'basket-weave' change.

**Management**

Dialysis and transplantation in chronic renal failure.

## Fabry's disease

**Aetiology**

X-linked inheritance. Glycosphingolipids deposited in many tissues including kidneys.

**Clinical features**

Haematuria, proteinuria, chronic renal failure.

**Pathology**

*LM.* Visceral epithelial cells of glomeruli show foamy swelling and endothelial and mesangial cells may show similar changes.
Progressive destruction of glomeruli.

**Management**

Transplantation of kidneys may replace deficient enzyme and restore normal function.

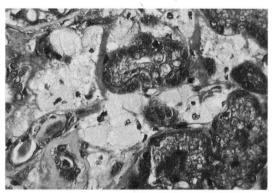

**Fig. 87** Interstitial foam cells in Alport's syndrome. (H & E × 80)

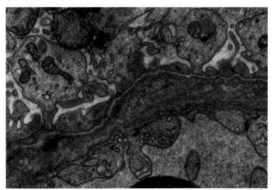

**Fig. 88** Irregularity of GBM with fibrillation in Alport's syndrome. (× 13 500)

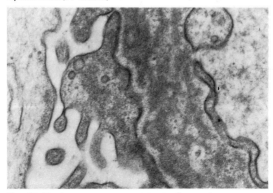

**Fig. 89** Basket-weave pattern in GBM in Alport's syndrome. (× 33 750)

# 26 | Acute Pyelonephritis

**Aetiology**

Invasion of the urinary tract including the renal interstitium by pathogenic organisms, most commonly *Escherichia coli.* Others include *Proteus, Klebsiella, Enterobacter, Pseudomonas* and *Staphylococcus aureus.* Predisposing factors include any structural abnormality (e.g. urinary tract obstruction, vesico-ureteric reflux, neurogenic bladder), foreign bodies (e.g. calculi and catheters) and systemic disturbance (e.g. diabetes mellitus). Common in women with normal renal tract, particularly in pregnancy.

**Clinical features**

General malaise and headache, nausea and vomiting. Fever and rigors. Dysuria, frequency, nocturia, haematuria, pyuria and unpleasant smell to urine. Pain and tenderness in suprapubic and renal (loin) areas. In rare cases septicaemia occurs resulting in endotoxic shock. There may be no symptoms (covert bacteruria).
*Investigation.* Important to obtain mid-stream urine to avoid contamination with skin flora. Microscopy reveals many pus cells and gram-stain shows bacteria (usually gram-negative rods). Culture reveals growth of bacteria. Significant growth is greater than $10^5$ organisms per ml.
Nature of organism is identified plus sensitivity to antibiotics.

**Pathology**

In a severe infection the swollen kidney may be studded with yellowish microabscesses.
*LM.* There is invasion of parenchyma by focal collections of polymorphs especially in cortex. Many tubules and collecting ducts are packed with polymorphs. Glomeruli are unaffected.

**Management**

Appropriate antibiotic, e.g. ampicillin or cotrimoxazole, depending upon sensitivities. Longterm suppressive therapy may be required in patients with recurrent infection. Good fluid intake and appropriate analgesia.

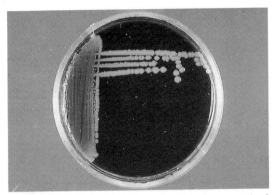

**Fig. 90** Culture of mid stream urine showing growth of *E. coli.*

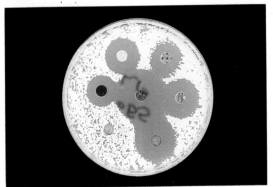

**Fig. 91** Culture plate with antibiotic discs showing sensitivity to antibiotics.

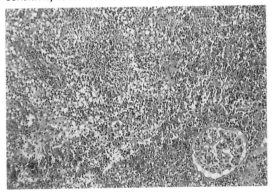

**Fig. 92** Intense tubulo-interstitial infiltrate of polymorphs. Glomerulus is spared. (H & E × 80)

**Aetiology**

Incompetence of the sphincter at the junction of the ureter with the bladder. Majority primary and are present at birth. Unilateral or bilateral. When micturition occurs urine refluxes back up the ureter (vesico-ureteric reflux), and occasionally into the kidney (intra-renal reflux) via ducts of Bellini. Recurrent urinary tract infections occur with scarring of the kidney.

**Clinical features**

In childhood recurrent urinary tract infection is common. If reflux is minimal there is often spontaneous cure. If the reflux is severe there is progressive shrinking and scarring of the kidneys which, if bilateral, results in chronic renal failure. Investigation is aimed at demonstration of the reflux of opaque medium from the bladder into the ureters and kidney during micturition (voiding cystourethrogram).

**Pathology**

The kidney shows coarse scarring, often maximal at the poles and a variable degree of pelvi-calyceal dilatation. Calyces underlying cortical scars always show dilatation.
*LM.* Initially there will be focal fibrous scarring but progressive fibrosis, chronic inflammation and tubular atrophy herald the onset of renal failure. Glomeruli are initially spared but later become sclerosed. At this stage the vascular changes of hypertension will be present.

**Management**

Treat recurrent urinary infections with appropriate antibiotic. Surgery in childhood if reflux severe before renal damage occurs.

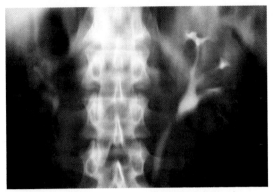

**Fig. 93** Intravenous urogram showing unilateral shrunken right kidney.

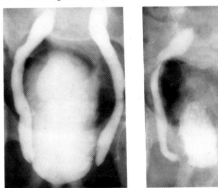

**Fig. 94** Voiding cystourethrogram showing reflux of contrast up ureter on voiding.

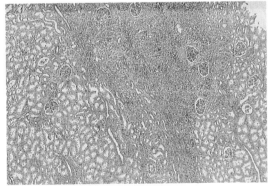

**Fig. 95** Wedge-shaped radial scar in reflux nephropathy. (H & E × 32)

## 28 | Chronic Renal Infection

### Chronic pyelonephritis

**Aetiology**

Recurrent urinary tract infections in the presence of obstruction, calculi or vesico-ureteric reflux.

**Clinical features**

May be recurrent urinary infection over a number of years. Eventually symptoms of chronic renal failure occur. Urine culture may reveal recurrent infection. Intravenous urogram shows small shrunken scarred kidneys with 'clubbed' calyces.

**Pathology**

The kidneys are irregularly scarred, often at the poles.
*LM.* A chronic inflammatory infiltrate in a fibrotic interstitium with tubular atrophy. Glomerular hyalinisation and arterial narrowing are found in long-standing cases.

**Management**

Appropriate antibiotics, either repeated or longterm. Chronic renal failure as appropriate.

### Renal tuberculosis

**Clinical features**

Cystitis, haematuria, pyuria.
Early morning urine samples—culture for tubercle bacilli and stain for acid and alcohol fast bacilli. Hydronephrosis and chronic renal failure may occur.

**Pathology**

Tubercles occur throughout the kidneys and large cavitating lesions develop in the medulla.

**Management**

Anti-tuberculous drugs.

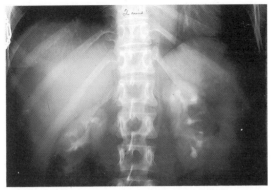

**Fig. 96** Intravenous urogram showing small shrunken scarred kidneys with clubbed calyces.

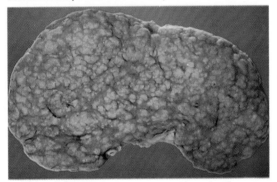

**Fig. 97** Cortex shows coarse scarring in chronic pyelonephritis.

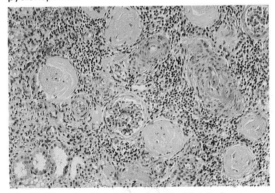

**Fig. 98** Many hyalinised glomeruli with tubular atrophy and chronic inflammation. (H & E × 80)

# 29 | Acute Interstitial Nephritis

**Aetiology**

This is an acute condition causing renal failure in which there is no glomerular pathology but with an interstitial response described below, caused by a variety of agents including antibiotics (penicillin, methicillin, cephalosporins, rifampicin and sulphonamides), diuretics (frusemide and thiazides), allopurinol, phenytoin, phenindione, and phenylbutazone.

**Clinical features**

Usually presents with acute renal failure.

**Pathology**

*LM.* The predominant finding is of an intense interstitial infiltrate of chronic inflammatory cells, lymphocytes, histiocytes and plasma cells which may be focal or diffuse in the cortex. Where eosinophils are seen within the infiltrate this suggests drug-associated hypersensitivity. There is usually interstitial oedema and foci of tubular disruption can be identified. Glomeruli and blood vessels are not damaged and, as this is an acute onset and mostly recoverable lesion, fibrosis is not an important feature.
*IF.* In a few cases linear staining of tubular basement membranes with IgG and C3 can be seen.

**Management**

Withdrawal of toxic agent, appropriate treatment for acute renal failure, and steroids.

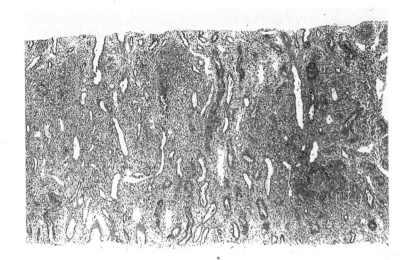

**Fig. 99** Needle biopsy showing intense, inflammatory infiltrate. (H & E × 45)

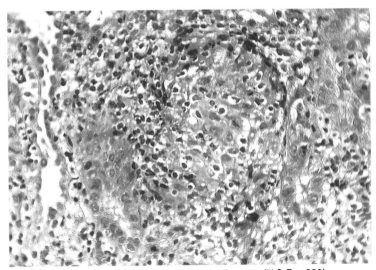

**Fig. 100** Inflammatory destruction of tubules is seen. (H & E × 280)

# 30 | Analgesic Nephropathy

**Aetiology**

Excessive intake of phenacetin and aspirin affect blood supply to renal papillae causing necrosis.

**Clinical features**

Mostly affects women, age range 40–50 and older men. Early symptoms include haematuria, sterile pyuria and polyuria. Acute renal failure can occur when separated papillae obstruct the ureters. Often associated with urinary tract infection. Many cases progress to chronic renal failure. The disease occurs most commonly in countries such as Switzerland and Australia where the analgesic intake is high (social habit). In these areas it is a significant cause of end-stage renal failure.
There is an association between high analgesic intake and transitional cell carcinoma of the renal pelvis.

**Pathology**

Kidneys may be of normal size or show some reduction with cortical scarring. Necrotic papillae are usually yellow or pale brown and may contain foci of calcification.
*LM.* The necrotic papilla shows ghostly remnants of ducts with little or no inflammatory infiltrate. A variable background of chronic interstitial nephritis affects the cortex secondary to papillary necrosis.

**Management**

Stop analgesics. Control infection. Appropriate renal failure treatment.

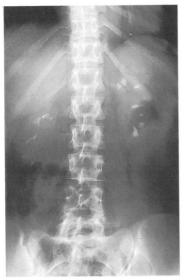

**Fig. 101** Straight X-ray showing papillary calcification and small kidneys.

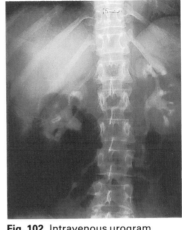

**Fig. 102** Intravenous urogram showing papillae separated from medulla—'signet ring' appearance.

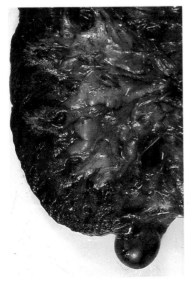

**Fig. 103** Pale zones delineate necrotic papillae.

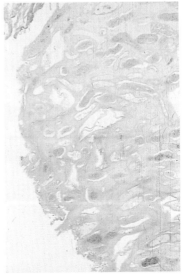

**Fig. 104** Ghostly remnants of ducts in a necrotic papilla. (H & E × 32)

# 31 | Renal Tubular Acidosis

**Aetiology**

Reduced ability of renal tubules to excrete acid. Type 1 (distal tubular) inherited as autosomal dominant. Distal tubules fail to secrete hydrogen and ammonium ions. Also decreased concentrating ability, and increased potassium and calcium excretion.

Type 2 (proximal tubules) usually hereditary. Generalised proximal tubule dysfunction. Bicarbonate reabsorption in the proximal tubule is deficient, results in metabolic acidosis, and moderate increase in calcium and potassium urinary excretion.

**Clinical features**

Growth affected with rickets because of calcium loss. Renal stones and nephrocalcinosis occur. Biochemical tests show metabolic acidosis with low plasma bicarbonate, hyperchloraemia, hypokalaemia, hypocalcaemia. A urinary acidification test should be performed. Ammonium chloride 0.1 g/kg body weight is given orally. This is broken down by the liver to release hydrogen ions in the blood which should be excreted by the kidney. Urine pH and urinary excretion of ammonium, acid, and bicarbonate are measured.

Patients with Type 1 distal RTA are unable to lower urine pH to $< 5.5$ and urinary ammonium, acid and bicarbonate are low.

In Type 2 RTA the urine pH can be lowered to $< 5.5$, ammonium and acid excretion may be normal and bicarbonate may or may not be present in the urine.

**Management**

Sodium bicarbonate and potassium citrate.

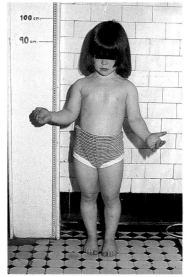

**Fig. 105** Patient aged 8 years with renal tubular acidosis showing stunting of growth.

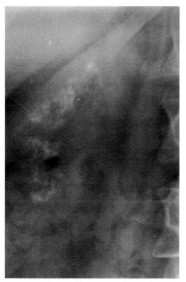

**Fig. 106** Straight X-ray of renal tract showing nephrocalcinosis in patient with renal tubular acidosis.

## 32 | Fanconi Syndrome

**Aetiology**

Inherited—autosomal recessive. Acquired in cystinosis, glycogen storage disease, and exposure to toxic substances (an adult idiopathic form occurs). There is failure to resorb amino acids, sodium, potassium, calcium, phosphate, bicarbonate, glucose and proteins.

**Pathology**

In the inherited variety there is a 'swan neck' deformity of the first part of the proximal tubule.

**Clinical features**

Dwarfism, rickets.
Blood tests reveal a low plasma calcium, phosphate, sodium, potassium and bicarbonate.
Renal failure rarely develops.
The prognosis in the acquired form, e.g. cystinosis, is poor, but in the adult form (idiopathic) is good if appropriate treatment is given.

**Management**

Fluids, sodium, potassium, phosphate and bicarbonate supplements.

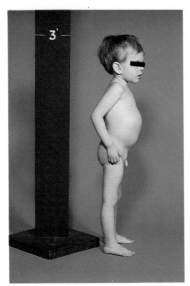

**Fig. 107** Child aged 8 years with dwarfism due to Fanconi syndrome secondary to cystinosis.

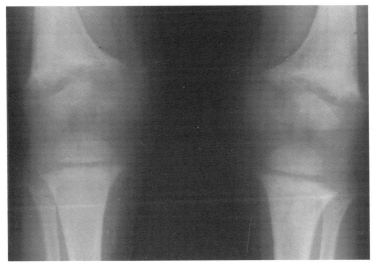

**Fig. 108** X-ray of patient with Fanconi syndrome showing rickets.

## 33 | Nephrogenic Diabetes Insipidus

**Aetiology**

An inability of the kidneys to respond to circulating anti-diuretic hormone (normal or increased levels).
*a.* Inherited.
*b.* Acquired: chronic renal disease, urinary tract obstruction, following tubular necrosis, renal transplantation, potassium deficiency, hypercalcaemia, drugs, e.g. lithium.

**Clinical features**

Polyuria, thirst and polydipsia (excessive drinking).
*Investigations.* Plasma and urine osmolality are measured after fluid withdrawal and after the administration of vasopressin.
1. Withdraw fluid from 6 pm on Day 1.
2. Hourly urine samples from 6 am–11 am on Day 2 for osmolality. Normally increase to > 900 mmol/kg of water. Patients with NDI show little rise beyond 300 mmol/kg.
3. Plasma osmolality at 11 am (should be > 288 mosmol/kg). Patients with pituitary diabetes insipidus show a rise of urine osmolality to > 600 mosmol/kg. Patients with NDI show no rise.
4. At 11 am give 5 units aqueous Pitressin subcutaneously.
5. Urine osmolality on hourly sample at 12 noon. Patients with NDI show no rise.

**Management**

ADH is of no value. Diuretics should be tried; they cause a fall in GFR and enhance absorption of fluid in the proximal tubule.

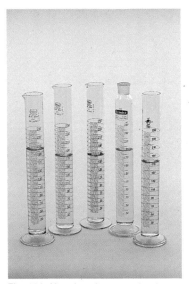

**Fig. 109** Hourly urine samples for osmolality from 6 am–11 am in patient with nephrogenic diabetes insipidus (polyuria).

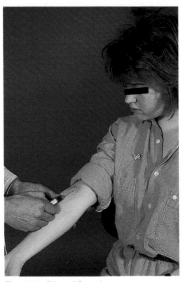

**Fig. 110** Blood for plasma osmolality at 11 am.

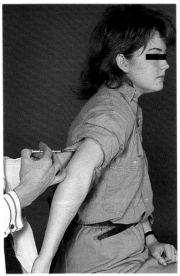

**Fig. 111** Injection of 4 units aqueous Pitressin at 11 am.

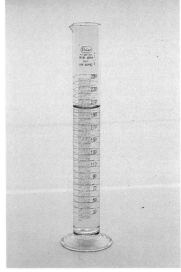

**Fig. 112** Urine osmolality at 12 midday (polyuria persists).

# 34 | Polycystic Renal Disease

**Aetiology**

Infantile and childhood: autosomal recessive, rare.
Adult: autosomal dominant.
Genetic markers are of use in early diagnosis with HLA association.

**Clinical features**

*Infantile.* At birth poor renal function leads to death within days from renal failure.
*Childhood.* Shows less renal failure; death from portal hypertension and liver failure.
*Adult.* May be asymptomatic.
Often haematuria, abdominal pain and hypertension.
Many cases progress to chronic renal failure.
*Investigations.* X-ray renal tract and intravenous urogram. Ultrasound of kidneys very helpful.

**Pathology**

*Infantile.* Bilateral: kidneys greatly enlarged but retain smooth renal outline. Cysts are found throughout cortex and medulla.
Always associated with intrahepatic cystic disease and fibrosis.
*Adult.* Bilateral: kidneys often huge and diffusely filled with bulging cysts containing clear fluid or blood. Normal renal tissue gradually compressed and hypertensive changes and glomerulosclerosis occur. There may be hepatic cysts in 30 % of cases.

**Management**

Analgesia for pain.
Appropriate renal failure treatment.
Genetic counselling.

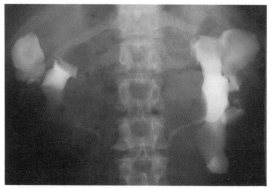

**Fig. 113** IVU showing displacement of calyces by multiple cysts in polycystic renal disease.

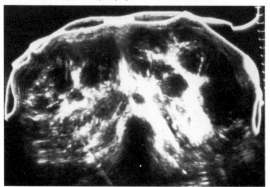

**Fig. 114** Ultrasound showing multiple cysts in both kidneys.

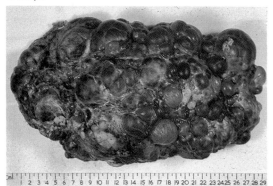

**Fig. 115** Adult polycystic disease: enlarged kidney with multiple cysts.

# 35 | Renal Calculi

**Aetiology**

Due to precipitation of calcium oxalate or calcium phosphate or both (80 %), uric acid (5 %), cystine (1 %), struvite—magnesium ammonium phosphate (14 %).
Precipitation is encouraged by:
Supersaturation (either dehydration or increased concentration of e.g. calcium oxalate in hypercalcaemic states; uric acid in gout) or pH changes, e.g. cystine and uric acid precipitate in acid urine.
Absence of inhibitors, e.g. inorganic pyrophosphate.
Infections: particularly struvite stones with proteus.

**Clinical features**

May by asymptomatic if in renal parenchyma or immobile in renal pelvis.
Renal calculi encourage recurrent urinary tract infection.
Haematuria.
Renal colic: severe pain in loin radiating to groin and genitalia, when calculi travel down ureter.
Obstruction and hydronephrosis if stone stationary in ureter.
Renal failure acute or chronic if persistent obstruction (bilateral), or associated infection.

*Investigations*
Serum and urinary calcium—idiopathic hypercalcaemia or hyperparathyroidism.
Serum and urine urate—gout.
Urine cystine.
Urine acidification test—RTA.
Urine culture.
Plain X-ray and IVU.
Cystoscopy and retrograde pyelography.

**Management**

Pain relief.
High fluid intake.
Antibiotics if infection.
Surgery if obstruction or recurrent infection.
Lithotripter can be used to break up calculi by non-invasive technique.

NEPHROLOGY

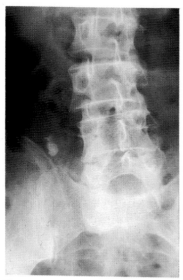

**Fig. 116** Plain X-ray showing stone in line of left ureter.

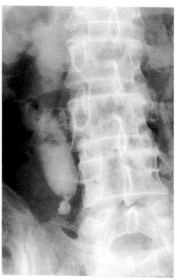

**Fig. 117** Intravenous urogram showing obstruction of contrast due to stone in left ureter.

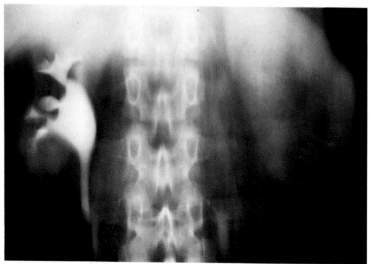

**Fig. 118** Intravenous urogram showing left kidney nephrographic phase due to obstruction.

## 36 | Urinary Tract Obstruction

**Aetiology**

Affecting urethra, bladder or ureter(s). Maybe acute or chronic. Caused by urethral valves, bladder neck obstruction, uretero-vesical and pelvi-ureteric abnormalities, prostatic hypertrophy, calculi, blood clots, sloughed papillae.
Tumour: intrinsic, e.g. bladder carcinoma, or extrinsic, e.g. carcinoma cervix, prostate.
Retroperitoneal fibrosis.
Neurological defects, i.e. neurogenic bladder, spinal cord lesions.

**Clinical features**

Acute obstruction. Pain due to retention of urine in either bladder or renal pelvis. The bladder is distended in urethral obstruction. Clinical examination may often reveal the cause, e.g. enlarged prostate on rectal examination or cervical tumour on vaginal examination. Hydronephrotic kidneys can be palpated on bimanual examination.
Chronic obstruction leads to renal failure which becomes permanent if obstruction not relieved.
*Investigation.* Ultrasound of the urinary tract. Straight X-ray (stones) or intravenous urogram. Cystoscopy for bladder lesions and retrograde pyelography for definition of ureteric lesions.

**Pathology**

If obstruction for more than a few hours hydronephrosis occurs; bilateral if obstruction at bladder outlet or bilateral ureteric lesions. Chronic obstruction causes atrophy of renal parenchyma.

**Management**

If urethral, a catheter should be passed.
Surgical management often required.
Renal failure management.

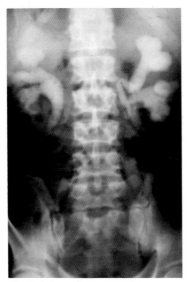

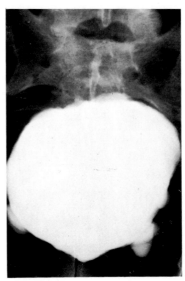

**Fig. 119** Intravenous urogram
showing bilateral hydronephrosis.

**Fig. 120** Intravenous urogram
showing large distended bladder
due to bladder neck obstruction.

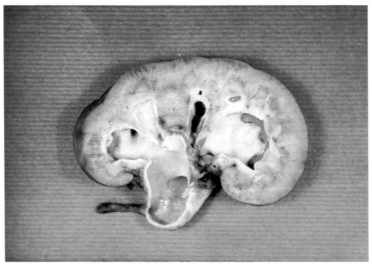

**Fig. 121** Dilated pelvis and calyces due to pelvi-ureteric obstruction.

# 37 | Renal Artery Stenosis

**Aetiology**

Atheroma males and females. Fibromuscular dysplasia most common in females in third and fourth decades.

**Clinical features**

May be asymptomatic and does not always cause hypertension. However a small percentage (1–5 %) of patients with hypertension have renal artery stenosis. Pointers to this aetiology in hypertensive patients are relative youth and resistance to anti-hypertensive treatment. There may be a bruit in the flank. The intravenous urogram shows a small kidney with a delay in the appearance of contrast medium. A radionuclide hippuran renogram shows a delayed vascular phase. A renal arteriogram is necessary to make the definitive diagnosis.

**Pathology**

Fibromuscular dysplasia displays a variety of patterns but commonly shows both narrowed and dilated segments due to irregular foci of fibromuscular hypertrophy. This may be bilateral and affects renal artery and main branches. Ischaemic changes are often found in the affected kidney and in some, hyperplasia of the JGA is a feature.

**Management**

Medical treatment alone can be tried. Surgical correction of the stenosis is effective but not without risk. The percutaneous dilatation of the stenosis by balloon catheter does not require surgical intervention or general anaesthesia and is proving effective in relieving the stenosis and curing hypertension in a proportion of cases.

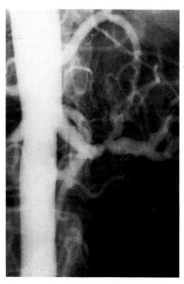

**Fig. 122** Renal arteriogram: fibro-muscular dysplasia with typical 'beaded' appearance of renal arteries.

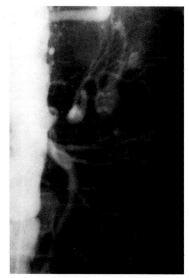

**Fig. 123** Renal arteriogram showing localised stenosis in renal artery due to atheroma.

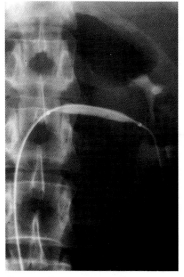

**Fig. 124** Percutaneous dilatation of renal artery stenosis using balloon catheter in stenosed segment of renal artery.

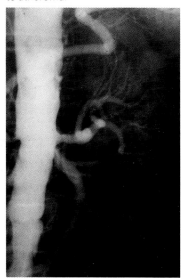

**Fig. 125** Renal arteriogram of renal artery stenosis after dilatation.

## Urinary Tract Infections (UTI)

Asymptomatic bacteruria occurs in 5 % and symptomatic UTI in 1−2 % of pregnant patients.

## Acute Renal Failure

**Aetiology**

*a.* Septic abortion.
*b.* Bleeding complications, especially placental abruption.

**Pathology**

There may be acute tubular necrosis or infarction of the cortex of both kidneys (focal to subtotal).

## Chronic Renal Failure

**Aetiology**

Idiopathic post-partum (2−3 w) renal failure.

**Pathology**

*LM.* Intimal thickening in interlobular arteries and arterioles and fibrin may be present. Glomeruli show areas of necrosis and diffuse thickening of capillary walls. *EM.* The glomerular capillary wall thickening is due to subendothelial accumulation of finely granular material which is probably related to fibrin deposition.

## Hypertension Disorders

A major cause of morbidity and death to mother and foetus.
1. *Pre-eclampsia* (hypertension, proteinuria and oedema) in last trimester.
2. *Chronic hypertension*, either essential or secondary, found in early pregnancy.

**Pathology**

*LM.* The glomeruli are enlarged showing marked swelling of endothelial cytoplasm and some mesangial prominence. *EM.* The capillary lumina are filled with vacuolar blebs of endothelial cytoplasm and platelets and fibrin can also be found.

**Management**

Rest, anti-hypertensive therapy, delivery of baby.

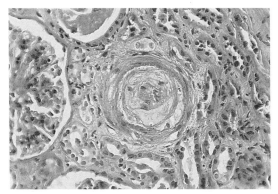

**Fig. 126** Post-partum renal failure: arterial occlusion due to sub-intimal thickening. (H & E × 200)

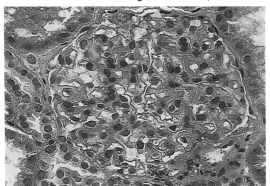

**Fig. 127** Pre-eclampsia: glomerulus showing endothelial swelling. (H & E × 320)

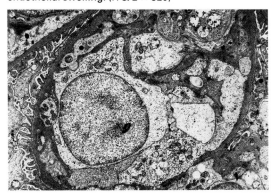

**Fig. 128** Marked endothelial swelling all but obliterates the lumen. (× 3 375)

# 39 | Hypertension and the Kidney (1)

A patient with hypertension may fall into one of the following 3 categories.
1. Benign hypertension, with secondary changes in the kidney.
2. Malignant hypertension with aggressive seconday changes in the kidney.
3. Renal conditions causing secondary hypertension.

## Benign essential hypertension

**Aetiology**

Remains obscure. Possible disturbance in relationship between sodium balance, hormones (renin, angiotensin, aldosterone, prostaglandins, natriuretic factor), cardiac output, peripheral resistance, and neurogenic mechanisms.

**Clinical features**

No specific symptoms of hypertension itself. Increased risk of cardiac failure, myocardial infarction, cerebral haemorrhage or thrombosis and malignant hypertension. The risk of significant nephrosclerosis is small (2–5 %) but progression to chronic renal failure is higher with severe uncontrolled hypertension, e.g. levels of 220/120.

**Pathology**

Both kidneys are usually reduced in size and uniform, fine scarring of cortex results in granular contraction of the kidney.
*LM.* Arteries show intimal thickening while arterioles show hyaline thickening of their media. Tubular atrophy and interstitial fibrosis can be found and glomerular hyalinisation is seen in long-standing cases.

**Management**

Anti-hypertensive drugs, e.g. diuretics, beta-blockers, calcium channel blockers.

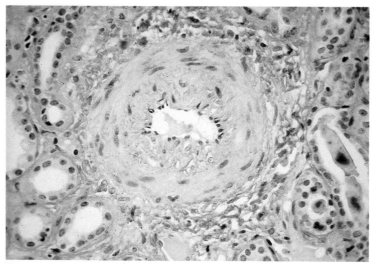

**Fig. 129** Benign hypertension: arteriosclerosis. (MSB & 280)

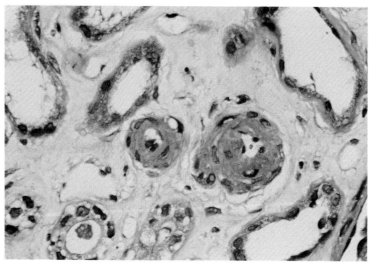

**Fig. 130** Benign hypertension: arteriolar hyalinisation and interstitial fibrosis. (H & E × 280)

| # Hypertension and the Kidney (2)

## Malignant hypertension

**Aetiology**

Severe uncontrolled hypertension leads to pathophysiological mechanisms affecting arterioles throughout the body, disturbances in vascular permeability mediated by hormones (possibly angiotensin or prostaglandin), and activation of clotting mechanisms similar to disseminated intravascular coagulation.

**Clinical features**

1. Very high blood pressure, e.g. 240/140.
2. Retinopathy. Fluffy exudates and flame haemorrhages. The above 2 abnormalities constitute malignant hypertension (WHO classification). The renal features include haematuria, and deterioration of renal function progressing to chronic renal failure. Progression leads to papilloedema, encephalopathy, coma and death.

**Pathology**

The cortical surface usually shows petechial haemorrhages.
*LM.* Fibrinoid necrosis of arterioles is the hallmark of the malignant phase while arteries, mainly interlobular, show intimal proliferation of layers of myxoid and collagenous material. Glomeruli frequently show areas of fibrinoid necrosis and there can be a marked proliferation of cells both intraglomerular and those lining Bowman's capsule.

**Management**

Intensive anti-hypertensive therapy often by intravenous route.

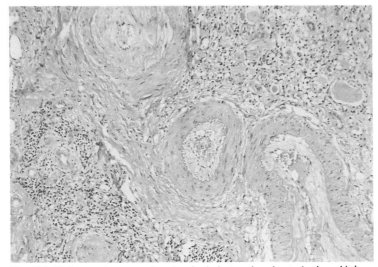

**Fig. 131** Malignant hypertension: luminal obstruction due to 'onion-skin' thickening of sub-intima. (H & E × 40)

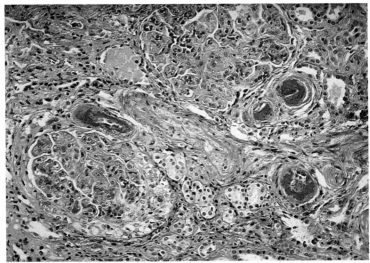

**Fig. 132** Malignant hypertension: arteriolar fibrinoid necrosis. (H & E × 112)

# Hypertension and the Kidney (3)

## Hypertension secondary to renal disease

**Aetiology**

A combination of salt and fluid retention and hormonal (renin-angiotensins-aldosterone) disturbance occurring in:
1. Various forms of glomerular nephritis.
2. Renovascular disease.
3. Chronic renal failure.
4. Pregnancy.
5. Renal transplant rejection.

**Clinical features**

The features of the particular renal disease are present (see appropriate section in text).
The hypertension is often severe and difficult to control. Severe uncontrolled hypertension leads to further renal damage and the syndrome of malignant hypertension may develop (see p. 89). Other features of hypertension (cardiac failure, myocardial infarction and cerebro-vascular accident) may occur.

**Pathology**

See appropriate section.

**Management**

Attention to primary renal disease.
Anti-hypertensive therapy—usually requires higher doses of drugs—e.g. diuretics, beta-blockers, or combinations, e.g. addition of calcium channel blocker (e.g. nifedipine) or vasodilator (e.g. prazosin or minoxidil).

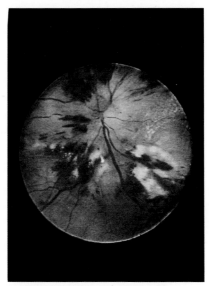

**Fig. 133** Fundus from patient with malignant hypertension showing exudates, haemorrhages and papilloedema.

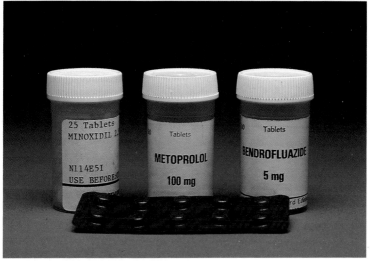

**Fig. 134** Multiple anti-hypertensive therapy in patient with hypertension associated with chronic renal failure.

## Aetiology

Acute renal failure is defined as a sudden fall in glomerular filtration rate, often with oliguria, with elevation of blood urea and creatinine, and often with metabolic acidosis and hyperkalaemia.

**Pre-renal failure**

This is due to circulatory insufficiency with a fall in renal blood flow and GFR.
1. *Hypovolaemia.* Haemorrhage, trauma, burns, electrolyte loss (vomiting), gastro-intestinal obstruction, severe diarrhoea, gastro-intestinal fistulae.
2. *Hypotension.* e.g. myocardial infarction, septicaemia.

**Renal (parenchymal) failure**

1. *Acute tubular necrosis.* (a) Ischaemic—occurs when factors causing pre-renal failure are prolonged or severe. (b) Nephrotoxic, e.g. heavy metals, organic solvents, sodium chlorate.
2. *Acute interstitial nephritis.* See p. 65.
3. *Glomerular disease.* (a) Crescentic GN. (b) Systemic lupus. (c) Polyarteritis nodosa.
4. *Haemolytic uraemic syndrome* and disseminated intravascular coagulation.
5. *Metabolic causes.* e.g. hyperuricaemia, myeloma.

**Post-renal failure (obstruction)**

This can be caused by calculi, dislodged papillae in analgesic nephropathy and blood clots.

**Pathology of acute tubular necrosis**

(a) *Ischaemic.* There is interstitial oedema with patchy inflammatory infiltrate. Tubular lesions consist of focal dilatation, membrane breaks and luminal casts of red cells, epithelial cells and debris. Mitoses in tubular epithelial cells indicate regeneration.
(b) *Nephrotoxic.* The proximal convoluted tubule shows marked epithelial degeneration with vacuolation, desquamation and necrosis. Interstitial oedema and infiltrate are seen.

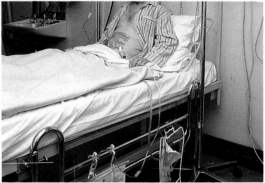

**Fig. 135** Patient with acute tubular necrosis following surgery associated with blood loss and septicaemia.

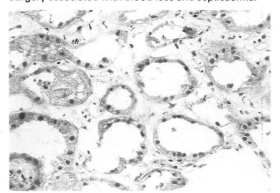

**Fig. 136** Tubules show basement membrane breaks. (H & E × 200)

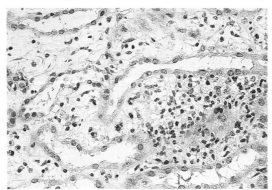

**Fig. 137** Interstitial oedema and inflammatory infiltrate. (H & E × 200)

## Clinical features

Patients with acute renal failure are often extremely ill.
It is important to identify (a) the features of renal failure, (b) the aetiological factors.

**Renal failure features**

*Fluid balance.* There is often oliguria (< 400 ml urine 24 h). Fluid overload may occur with peripheral and pulmonary oedema.
*Uraemia.* Nausea, vomiting, diarrhoea, drowsiness and coma may occur. The blood urea rises to high levels (40–80 mmol/l) within a few days. The bicarbonate level falls (metabolic acidosis).
*Potassium.* Hyperkalaemia is a dangerous condition and is increased by red cell destruction in haematoma or the gastro-intestinal tract and by hypoxia and acidosis. Levels above 6.5 mmol/l predispose to cardiac arrest (ventricular fibrillation).
*Infection.* Infection is a common complicating feature and carries a high mortality. It may occur in the lungs causing respiratory failure, any operative site, and in the blood (septicaemia).

**Aetiological factors**

*Pre-renal failure.* Circulatory failure or fluid depletion. Urine concentrated (> 600 mosmol/kg)
*Acute tubular necrosis.* Severe or prolonged circulatory failure or exposure to toxic agents. Urine isosmotic (250–350 mosmol/kg).
*Acute interstitial nephritis.* Exposure to toxic agents. Renal biopsy (see p. 65).
*Glomerular disease.* Nephritic illness, urine casts, red blood cells and protein. Renal biopsy.
*Haemolytic uraemic syndrome.* Purpura, bleeding, haemolysis thrombocytopenia, coagulation defects. Renal biopsy (see p. 55).
*Hyperuricaemia.* Tumour treatment.
*Post-renal (obstruction).* Calculi, or papillary necrosis. Radiology or ultrasound.

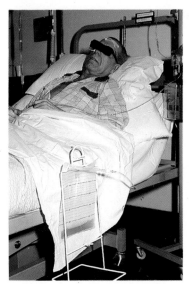

**Fig. 138** Patient with acute renal failure showing oliguria.

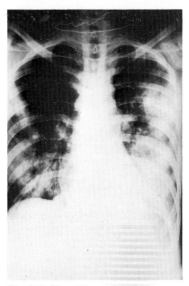

**Fig. 139** Chest X-ray showing bilateral broncho-pneumonia and fluid overload in patient with acute renal failure.

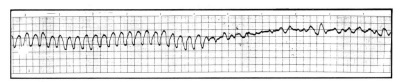

**Fig. 140** Electrocardiogram from patient with acute renal failure showing ventricular fibrillation due to hyperkalaemia.

## Management of renal failure

**Fluid**

500 ml (insensible loss) plus the negative fluid balance from the previous day (urine plus other fluid losses) should be given in a 24 h period. Oral or intravenous dextrose/saline. During recovery (diuretic phase) high fluid intake.

**Diet**

Patients often catabolic and require a high calorie intake (50 Kcal/Kg body weight). Slight reduction in dietary protein (40–50 g/24 h) may help to control uraemic features.

**Potassium**

If the blood potassium level is > 6 mmol/l, resonium 30 g orally or rectally. If this fails, glucose 50 ml of 50 % solution intravenously with soluble insulin 10 units.

**Dialysis**

If the above measures fail to control uraemic features, or if the blood urea rises above 40 mmol/l or the potassium above 6.5 mmol/l, dialysis in the form of haemodialysis or peritoneal dialysis should be instituted.

**Antibiotics**

Appropriate antibiotics should be given to control infection.

## Management of aetiological factors

*Pre-renal failure.*   Blood, fluid and electrolyte replacement. Inotropic agents for cardiac failure.
*Acute ischaemic tubular necrosis.*   As for pre-renal failure (central venous pressure line).
*Acute interstitial nephritis.*   Toxic agent withdrawn. Steroids.
*Glomerular disease.*   See appropriate sections in text.
*Haemolytic uraemic syndrome.*   See p. 55.
*Hyperuricaemia.*   Allopurinol and sodium bicarbonate.

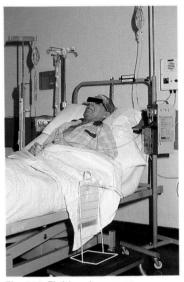

**Fig. 141** Fluid replacement controlled by central venous pressure line in patient with acute renal failure.

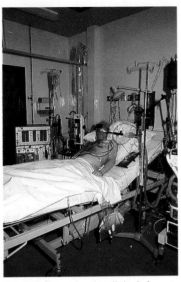

**Fig. 142** Acute haemodialysis in patient with acute renal failure.

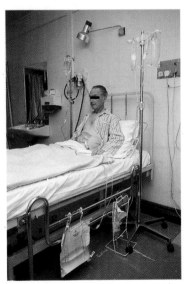

**Fig. 143** Acute peritoneal dialy in patient with acute renal failure.

## 41 | Chronic Renal Failure (1)

A clinical syndrome occurring at any age when renal function declines to low levels, usually over months or years.

**Aetiology**

Many of the conditions discussed in this book can lead to chronic renal failure. However, certain conditions have a high chance of progression.
1. Crescentic glomerulonephritis.
2. Membranous glomerulonephritis
3. Mesangiocapillary glomerulonephritis.
4. Focal glomerulosclerosis.
5. Diabetes mellitus.
6. Amyloidosis.
7. Reflux nephropathy/chronic pyelonephritis.
8. Polycystic renal disease.
9. Chronic obstructive renal disease.

**Clinical features**

Every system of the body can be affected. Skin: pigmentation, scratch marks, purpura, oedema, or dehydration. Cardio-vascular: hypertension, pericarditis. Respiratory: pulmonary oedema, and infection. Alimentary: vomiting, diarrhoea. Locomotor: osteodystrophy—bone pain, radiology, bone biopsy. Central nervous system: neuropathy, coma. Renal system: polyuria and features of primary disease, e.g. polycystic kidneys.

**Investigations**

Blood urea and creatinine elevated to high levels, e.g. 40 mmol/l and 900 $\mu$mol/l respectively. Metabolic acidosis with low bicarbonate, e.g. 8 mmol/l. Blood calcium may be reduced, alkaline phosphatase raised and radiological signs of renal osteodystrophy.
Normocytic, normochromic anaemia.
*Renal investigations.* Radiology or ultrasound show abnormal renal structure, e.g. polycystic kidneys or obstruction.
*Renal biopsy.* Should have been carried out in early stages of glomerulonephritic condition, e.g. crescentic glomerulonephritis. Little information gained once end-stage renal failure is reached.

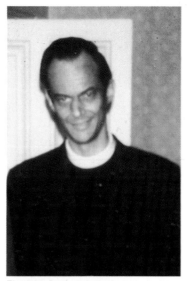

**Fig. 144** Patient with chronic renal failure showing pallor and general debility.

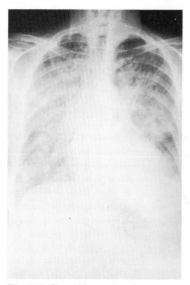

**Fig. 145** Chest X-ray showing pulmonary oedema in patient with chronic renal failure.

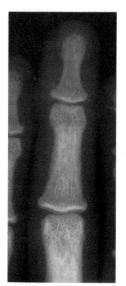

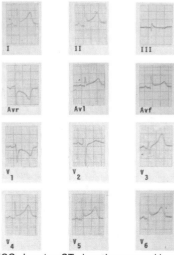

| | | |
|---|---|---|
| I | II | III |
| Avr | Avl | Avf |
| V₁ | V₂ | V₃ |
| V₄ | V₅ | V₆ |

**Fig. 147** ECG showing ST elevation caused by pericarditis in patient with chronic renal failure.

**Fig. 146** X-ray of phalanges showing renal osteodystrophy with subperiosteal erosions in patient with chronic renal failure.

## Conservative treatment

Treat the cause if possible, e.g. surgical treatment of obstruction.

**Fluids**

High fluid intake, up to 3 l daily until end-stage failure when oedema present, then:
1. Give diuretics often in high does, e.g. frusemide 500 mg daily.
2. Limit intake to control fluid overload, and accept elevation of blood urea and creatinine.

**Electrolyte intake**

Usually no sodium or potassium restriction until end-stage renal failure when may need to restrict. Sodium bicarbonate supplements 1−3 g/day for acidosis.

**Calories and protein**

Maintain nutrition with high carbohydrates and fat intake, 2000−2500 cal/day, plus low protein intake, 30−40 g/day.

**Anaemia**

Ferrous sulphate supplements but haemoglobin remains low, e.g. 6−7 g/dl. Blood transfusion should not be given unless severe anaemia ($< 5$ g/dl) or as part of blood transfusion protocol for renal transplantation.

**Hypertension**

Diuretics, beta blockers with care (reduced GFR), calcium channel blockers (e.g. nifedipine), minoxidil.

**Renal osteo-dystrophy**

Phosphate binder (e.g. Alucaps) to reduce plasma phosphate. One-alpha cholecalciferol to raise plasma calcium and heal or prevent osteodystrophy. Occasionally parathyroidectomy is required.

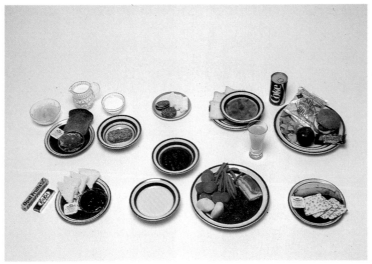

**Fig. 148** Day's supply of food showing low protein and high calorie content.

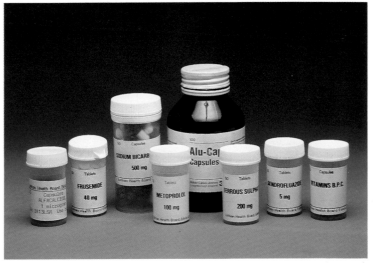

**Fig. 149** Medication consisting of ferrous sulphate, vitamin preparation, anti-hypertensive agents, phosphate binders and one-alfa cholecalciferol.

## Haemodialysis

When renal function is very poor (GFR < 5 ml/min), blood urea rises to > 40–50 mmol/l and creatinine to > 900–1000 $\mu$mol/l. Unless dialysis is instituted on a permanent basis, death of the patient will occur.

**Principles of haemodialysis**

The patient's blood is pumped through a cuprophane 'dialyser' which is surrounded by a physiological salt and glucose solution. Urea, creatinine, potassium and other toxic substances diffuse out of the blood through the cuprophane membrane into the dialysis solution.

**Practical aspects**

*Vascular access.* A good supply of blood must flow from the patient to the dialyser. The most usual method is via an arterio-venous fistula (Cimino-Brescia) created surgically in the arm. As an emergency procedure, an external arterio-venous (Quinton-Scribner) shunt at the wrist or ankle, or a double lumen subclavian catheter, can be used.
*Dialysis machine.* This consists of the electronic and mechanical components to pump blood safely to and from the patient, through the dialyser, and circulate dialysis fluid at the correct body temperature around the dialyser.
*Disposable items.* Fresh needles, blood lines and the dialyser are used on each occasion that the patient receives treatment.

**Procedures**

Needles are inserted into the arterio-venous fistula: one 'arterial' to take the blood from the patient to the dialyser, the other 'venous' to return blood to the patient.
Dialysis must be repeated 3 times per week, either in hospital, satellite unit or the patient's home.

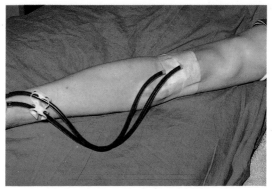

**Fig. 150** Arterio-venous Cimino fistula for vascular access in patient with chronic renal failure.

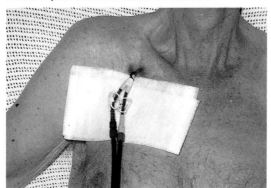

**Fig. 151** Double lumen sub-clavian line for vascular access in patient with chronic renal failure.

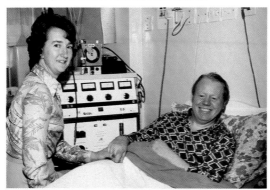

**Fig. 152** Patient on home dialysis in Portakabin.

## Continuous ambulatory peritoneal dialysis (CAPD)

**Principles**

Dialysis fluid placed in the peritoneal cavity is in contact with a large surface area of capillaries. Urea, creatinine, potassium and other toxic material diffuse out of the capillaries into the dialysis fluid which is drained away.

**Practical**

1. Access to the peritoneal cavity is via a permanent catheter (Tenckhoff) introduced through the abdominal wall.
2. Dialysis fluid is delivered from a 2 l bag via tubing connected to the peritoneal catheter using a sterile technique.
3. The dialysis fluid is left in the peritoneal cavity for 4–6 h, and the patient assumes normal ambulatory activities.
4. The dialysis fluid is then drained away and the cycle started again. Four cycles daily.
5. The above process is continued every day.

Most appropriate for elderly patients, those with vascular access problems, and diabetes.

Advantages: no machinery required, relatively cheap, avoidance of heparin and vascular access, removal of toxic substances (middle molecules), in diabetes insulin administered via peritoneal dialysis affording good control of blood glucose.

Disadvantages: no freedom from treatment and risk of peritonitis.

If recurrent peritonitis, efficiency of dialysis is lost and CAPD has to be abandoned.

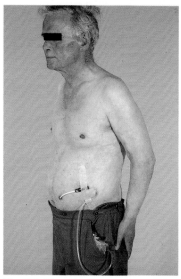

**Fig. 153** Tenckhoff intraperitoneal catheter.

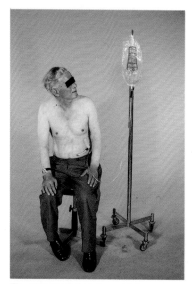

**Fig. 154** 2 l fluid infused into peritoneal cavity.

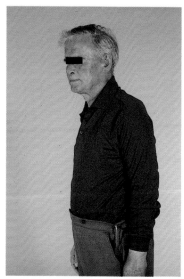

**Fig. 155** Patient mobile whilst dialysis continues via fluid in peritoneal cavity.

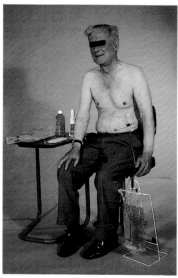

**Fig. 156** Drainage of fluid from peritoneal cavity 6 h later.

# Chronic Renal Failure (5)

## Renal transplantation

A functioning renal transplant is the 'ideal' treatment for chronic renal failure. Contra-indications include infection, e.g. tuberculosis, or urinary tract infection, malignancy, general debility, cardiac failure including ischaemic heart disease.

**Donor**

If possible a living related donor (twin, sibling or parent) is used (about 5–10 %). The majority are cadaver donors, mostly patients with severe head injury with 'brain-death', age 5–60 years, and with normal renal function.

**Matching**

ABO blood group matching is routine. All recipients have 'tissue-typing', i.e. HLA antigen status. Suitable donors are 'tissue-typed' and the best match obtained. There must be a negative cross-match between donor lymphocytes and recipient serum. In living related transplants the lymphocytes of the donor and recipient should not react (assessed by the mixed lymphocyte reaction, MLR).

**Surgery**

The kidney is positioned in the iliac fossa and the following anastomoses are made:
Donor renal artery to recipient hypogastric artery.
Donor renal vein to recipient external iliac vein.
Donor ureter to recipient bladder.

**Immuno-suppression**

Steroids (prednisolone), azathioprine, or cyclosporin. Blood transfusion prior to transplantation induces beneficial immunological events in the majority of recipients which leads to better transplant survival.

**Survival**

One year survival of 80–90 % can be expected with living donors, and 70–80 % with cadaver donors.

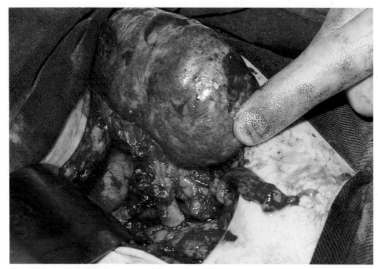

**Fig. 157** Surgical operation with placing of transplanted kidney in iliac fossa.

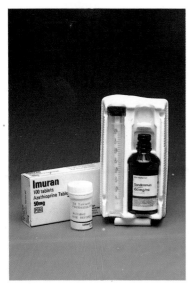

**Fig. 158** Medication to prevent rejection consisting of steroids, azathioprine and cyclosporin.

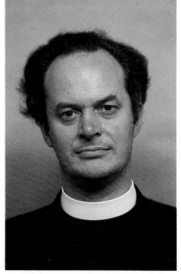

**Fig. 159** Renal transplant patient restored to normal health. (Same patient as Fig. 144.)

## Renal transplant rejection

**Aetiology**

Complex immunological mechanisms.

**Clinical features**

*Acute*
Fever, renal pain, oliguria, rapid increase in blood urea and creatinine.

*Chronic*
May be no symptoms. Gradual deterioration of renal function with proteinuria.

**Pathology**

The pathology of allograft rejection may be considered under three headings, hyperacute, acute and chronic rejection.

1. *Hyperacute rejection.* ABO mismatch or high titre of toxic antibodies to donor lymphocytes. Transplant capillaries and arterioles occluded by platelet thrombi and large numbers of polymorphs within an hour or two, leading to massive cortical necrosis.

2. *Acute rejection.* The tubules show foci of necrosis and the interstitium is oedematous and contains a marked infiltrate of macrophages and lymphocytes. Haemorrhage from peritubular capillaries may be seen. Glomeruli may show small thrombi and arterioles and interlobular arteries can show intimal swelling, or, in severe cases, fibrinoid necrosis.

3. *Chronic rejection.* The principal lesion affects arteries. The arcuate and interlobular arteries show luminal reduction due to accummulation of concentric layers of loosely cellular, subintimal material as a result of repeated deposition and incorporation of platelets and fibrin. Glomeruli frequently show mesangial matrix increase and irregular GBM thickening and there is a variable degree of tubular atrophy and interstitial fibrosis.

**Management**

High dose steroids.